Medite Diet Cookbook

50 Quick and Easy Recipes to Achieve a Healthier Lifestyle

By Harriet Bates

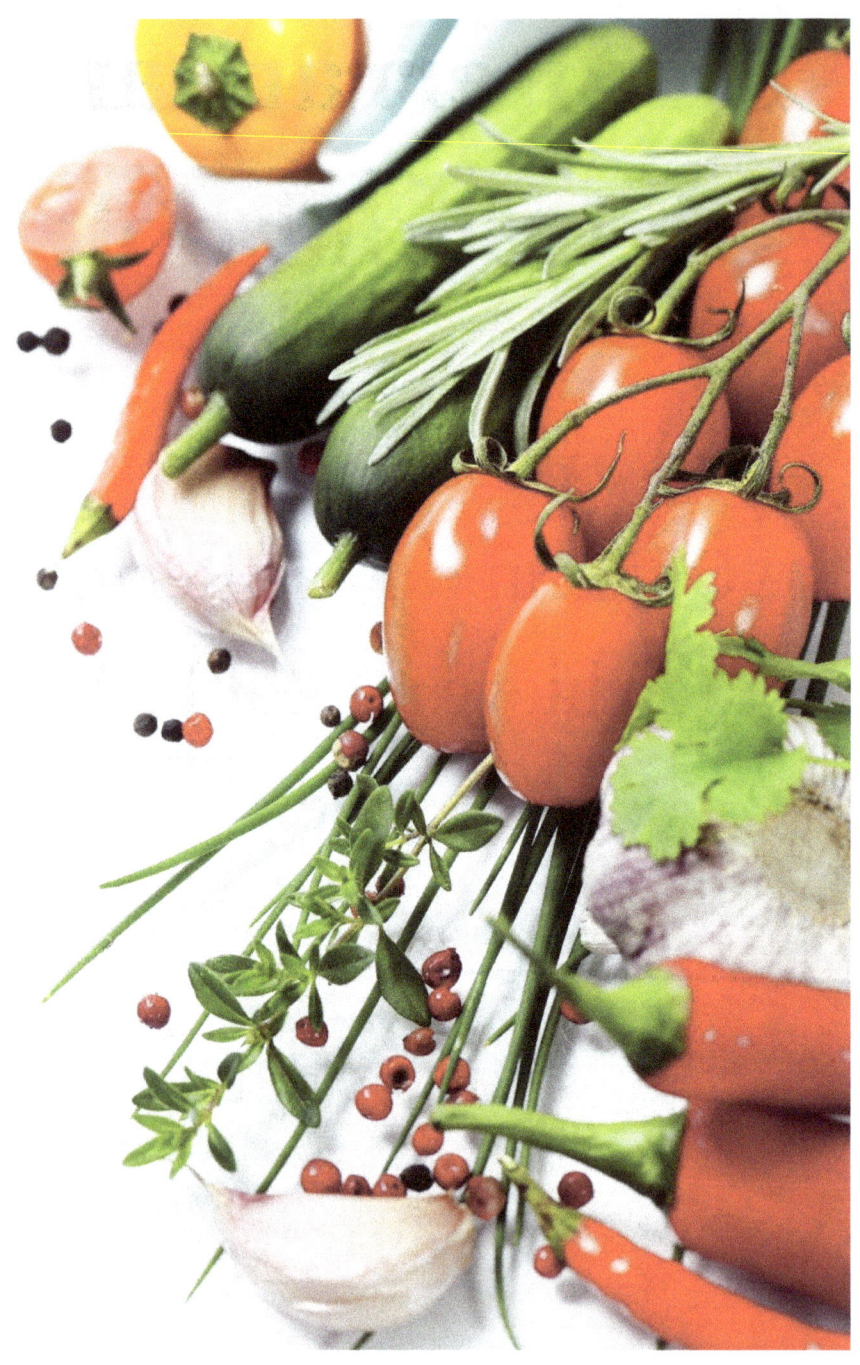

Table of Contents

Introduction **8**

Chapter 1: Breakfast and Snack Recipes **10**

    Avocado and Chickpea Sandwiches 11

    Raisin Quinoa Breakfast 13

    Banana Cinnamon Fritters 14

    Veggie Casserole 15

    Ground Beef and Brussels Sprouts 17

    Italian Mini Meatballs 18

    Mushroom and Olives Steaks 20

    Salmon Kebabs 21

    Mediterranean Baked Salmon 23

    Feta Cheese Baked in Foil 24

Chapter 2: Lunch & Dinner Recipes **25**

    Sausage and Beans Soup 27

    Jalapeno Grilled Salmon With Tomato Confit 29

    Chicken And Rice Soup 31

    Spicy Salsa Braised Beef Ribs 33

    Pork and Prunes Stew 35

Chapter 3: Meat Recipes **37**

    Pork And Figs Mix 39

Lamb Chops 41

Chicken Quinoa Pilaf 43

Greek Styled Lamb Chops 45

Bulgur And Chicken Skillet 46

Chapter 4: Poultry Recipes 48

Chicken And Spinach Cakes 49

Cream Cheese Chicken 51

Chicken And Lemongrass Sauce 53

Spiced Chicken Meatballs 55

Paprika Chicken Wings 57

Chapter 5: Fish and Seafood Recipes 59

Fried Salmon 61

Smoked Salmon And Veggies Mix 63

Berries And Grilled Calamari 64

Salmon And Zucchini Rolls 67

Scallions And Salmon Tartar 69

Chapter 6: Salads & Side Dishes 70

Instant Pot Collard Greens with Tomatoes 71

Instant Pot Millet Pilaf 73

Barley & Mushroom Soup 74

Instant Pot Stuffed Sweet Potatoes 76

Instant Pot Couscous and Vegetable Medley 78

Chickpea Pasta Salad 80

Bean Lettuce Wraps 82

Easy Lentil & Rice Bowl 84

Chickpea Pita Patties 86

Mushrooms with Soy Sauce Glaze 89

Cinnamon Quinoa Bars 91

Cucumber Olive Rice 93

Chicken And White Bean 95

Chorizo-kidney Beans Quinoa Pilaf 98

Belly-filling Cajun Rice & Chicken 100

Chapter 7: Dessert Recipes 102

Almonds And Oats Pudding 103

Chocolate Rice 104

Lemon And Semolina Cookies 106

Strawberry Sorbet 108

Halva (halawa) 110

Copyright 2021 by Harriet Bates - All rights reserved. The following Book is reproduced below with the goal of providing information that is as accurate and reliable as possible. Regardless, purchasing this Book can be seen as consent to the fact that both the publisher and the author of this book are in no way experts on the topics discussed within and that any recommendations or suggestions that are made herein are for entertainment purposes only. Professionals should be consulted as needed prior to undertaking any of the action endorsed herein.

This declaration is deemed fair and valid by both the American Bar Association and the Committee of Publishers Association and is legally binding throughout the United States.

Furthermore, the transmission, duplication, or reproduction of any of the following work including specific information will be considered an illegal act irrespective of if it is done electronically or in print. This extends to creating a secondary or tertiary copy of the work or a recorded copy and is only allowed with the express written consent from the Publisher. All additional right reserved.

The information in the following pages is broadly considered a truthful and accurate account of facts and as such, any inattention, use, or misuse of the information in question by the reader will render any resulting actions solely under their purview. There are no scenarios in which the publisher or the original author of this work can be in any fashion deemed liable for any hardship or damages that may befall them after undertaking information described herein.

Additionally, the information in the following pages is intended only for informational purposes and should thus be thought of as universal. As befitting its nature, it is presented without assurance regarding its prolonged validity or interim quality. Trademarks that are mentioned are done without written consent and can in no way be considered an endorsement from the trademark holder.

Introduction

Mediterranean diet is based on the eating habits of the inhabitants of the regions along the Mediterranean Sea, mostly from Italy, Spain and Greece; it is considered more a life style then a diet, in fact it also promotes physical activity and proper liquid (mostly water) consumption.

Depending on fresh seasonal local foods there are no strict rules, because of the many cultural differences, but there are some common factors.

Mediterranean diet has become famous for its ability to reduce heart disease and obesity, thanks to the low consumption of unhealthy fats that increase blood glucose.

Mediterranean diet is mostly plant based, so it's rich of antioxidants; vegetables, fruits like apple and grapes, olive oil, whole grains, herbs, beans and nuts are consumed in large quantities.

Moderate amounts of poultry, eggs, dairy and seafood are also common aliments, accompanied by a little bit of red wine (some studies say that in small amount it helps to stay healthy).

Red meat and sweets like cookies and cakes are accepted but are more limited in quantity.

Foods to avoid:

- refined grains, such as white bread and pasta
- dough containing white flour refined oils (even canola oil and soybean oil)
- foods with added sugars (like pastries, sodas, and candies)
- processed meats processed or packaged foods

Chapter 1: Breakfast and Snack Recipes

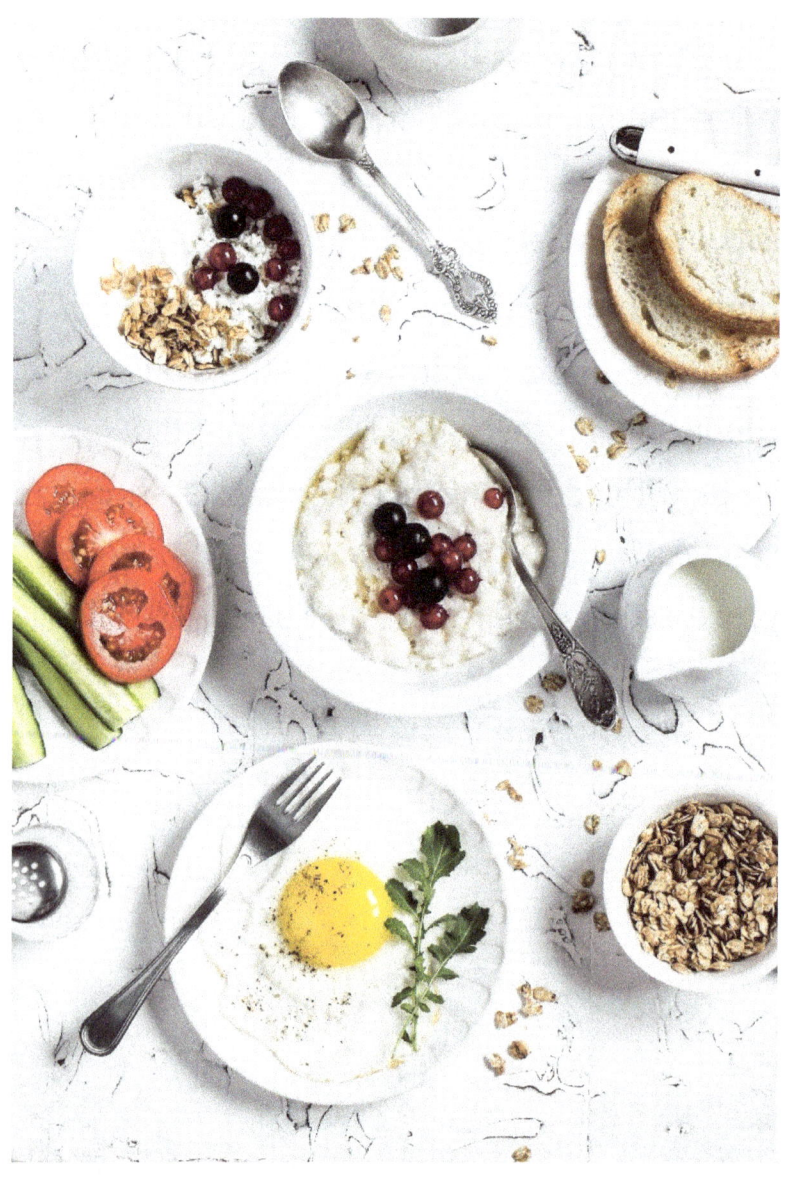

Avocado and Chickpea Sandwiches

Preparation: 4 min | Cooking: 0 minute| Servings: 4

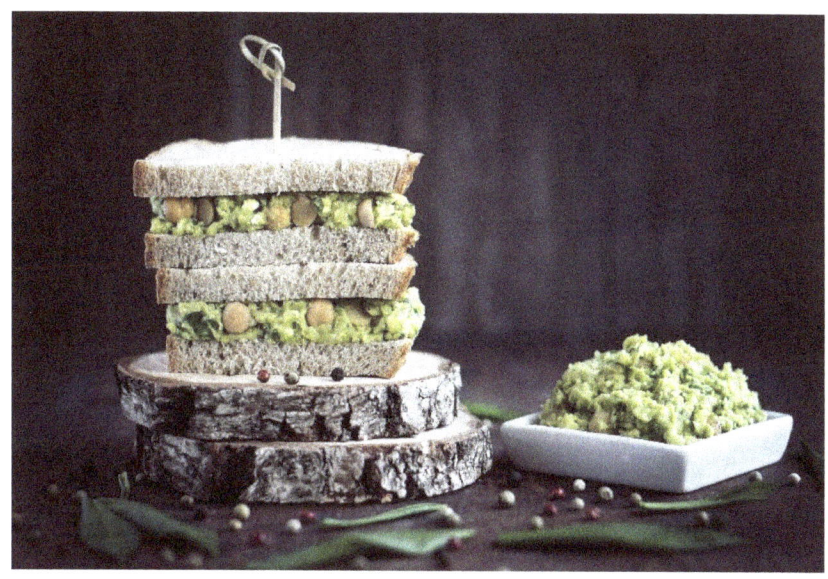

Ingredients

- 1/2 cup canned chickpeas
- 1 small avocado
- 2 green onions, finely chopped
- 1 egg, hard boiled
- 1/2 tomato, cucumber

Directions

1. Mash the avocado and chickpeas with a fork or potato masher until smooth. Add in green onions and salt and combine well.
2. Spread this mixture on the four slices of bread. Top each piece with tomato, cucumber and egg, and serve.

Nutrition: 309 calories; 9g fat; 2g protein

Raisin Quinoa Breakfast

Preparation: 15 min | Cooking: 0 minute| Servings: 4

Ingredients

- 1 cup quinoa
- 2 cups milk
- 2 tbsp. walnuts, crushed
- 2 tbsp. raisins, cranberries
- 1 tbsp. chia seeds

Directions

1. Rinse quinoa with cold water and drain. Place milk and quinoa into a saucepan and bring to a boil. Add ½ tsp. of vanilla. Adjust heat to low and simmer for 16 min stirring from time to time.
2. Set aside to cool then serve in a bowl, topped with honey, chia seeds, raisins, cranberries and crushed walnuts.

Nutrition: 299 calories; 7g fat; 1g protein

Banana Cinnamon Fritters

Preparation: 15 min | Cooking: 6 min | Servings: 4

Ingredients
- 1 cup self-rising flour
- 1 egg, beaten
- 3/4 cup sparkling water
- 2 tsp ground cinnamon
- 2-3 bananas, cut diagonally into 4 pieces each

Directions
1. Sift flour and cinnamon into a bowl and make a well in the center. Add egg and enough sparkling water to mix to a smooth batter.
2. Heat sunflower oil in a saucepan, enough to cover the base by 1-2 inch, so when a little batter dropped into the oil sizzles and rises to the surface.
3. Dip banana pieces into the batter, and then fry for 2-3 min or until golden. Pull out using slotted spoon and strain on paper towels. Sprinkle with sugar and serve hot.

Nutrition: 209 calories; 10g fat; 2g protein

Veggie Casserole

Preparation: 25 min | Cooking: 45 min | Servings: 4

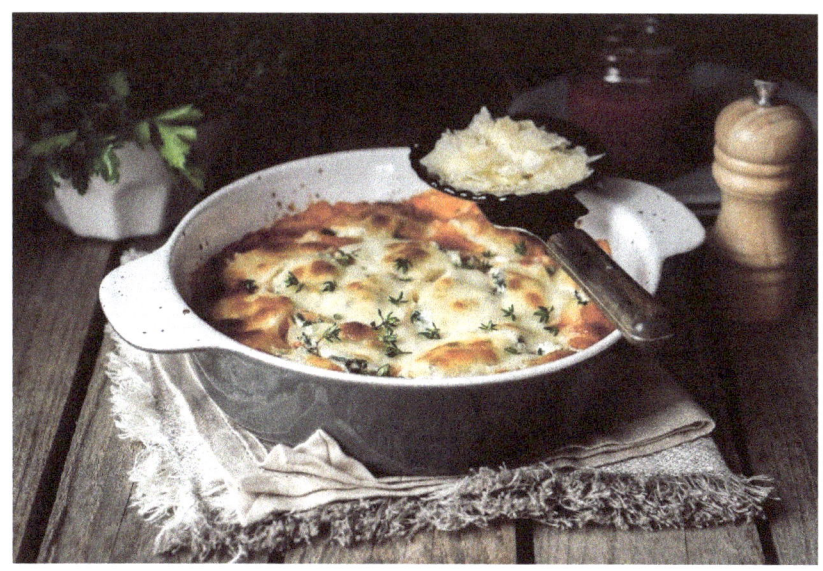

Ingredients

- 1 lb. okra, trimmed
- 3 tomatoes, cut into wedges
- 3 garlic cloves, chopped
- 1 cup fresh parsley leaves, finely cut

Directions

1. In a deep ovenproof baking dish, combine okra, sliced tomatoes, olive oil and garlic. Add in salt and black pepper to taste, and toss to combine.
2. Bake in a prepared oven at 350 F for 45 min. Garnish with parsley and serve.

Nutrition: 302 calories; 13g fat; 6g protein

Ground Beef and Brussels Sprouts

Preparation: 20 min | Cooking: 36 min | Servings: 4

Ingredients

- 6 oz. ground beef
- 2 garlic cloves, crushed
- ½ cup grated sweet potato
- 1 cup grated Brussels sprouts
- 1 egg, boiled

Directions

1. In a medium saucepan, cook olive oil over medium heat. Gently sauté the ½ onion and garlic until the onion is soft and translucent. Add in the beef and the sweet potato and cook until the meat is fully cooked.
2. Mix in the Brussels sprouts and cook for about 5 min more. Season well and serve topped with a boiled egg.

Nutrition: 314 calories; 15g fat; 6g protein

Italian Mini Meatballs

Preparation: 13 min | Cooking: 20 min | Servings: 6

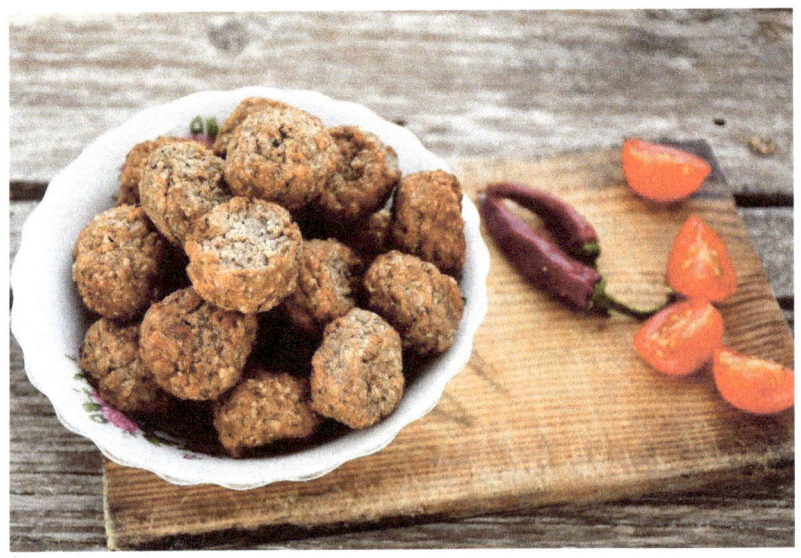

Ingredients

- 1 lb. ground beef
- 1 onion, grated
- 1 egg, lightly whisked
- 1 tsp garlic powder
- 1 tsp dried basil, oregano, parsley

Directions

1. Combine ground beef, onion, egg, parsley, garlic powder, basil and oregano. Mix very well with hands. Roll tablespoonful of the meat mixture into balls.
2. Place meatballs on a lined baking tray. Bake 20 min or until brown. Transfer to a serving plate and serve.

Nutrition: 275 calories; 9g fat; 1g protein

Mushroom and Olives Steaks

Preparation: 20 min | Cooking: 9 min | Servings: 6

Ingredients
- 1 lb. boneless beef sirloin steak
- 1 large onion, sliced
- 5-6 white mushrooms
- 1/2 cup green olives, coarsely chopped
- 1 cup parsley leaves, finely cut

Directions
1. Cook olive oil in a heavy bottomed pan at medium-high heat. Cook the steaks until well browned on each side then keep aside.
2. Gently sauté the onion in the same pan, for 3 min. Cook the mushrooms and olives until the mushrooms are done.
3. Situate the steaks back to the skillet, and cook for 5-6 min. Stir in parsley and serve.

Nutrition: 281 calories; 14g fat; 3g protein

Salmon Kebabs

Preparation: 30 min | Cooking: 6 min | Servings: 5

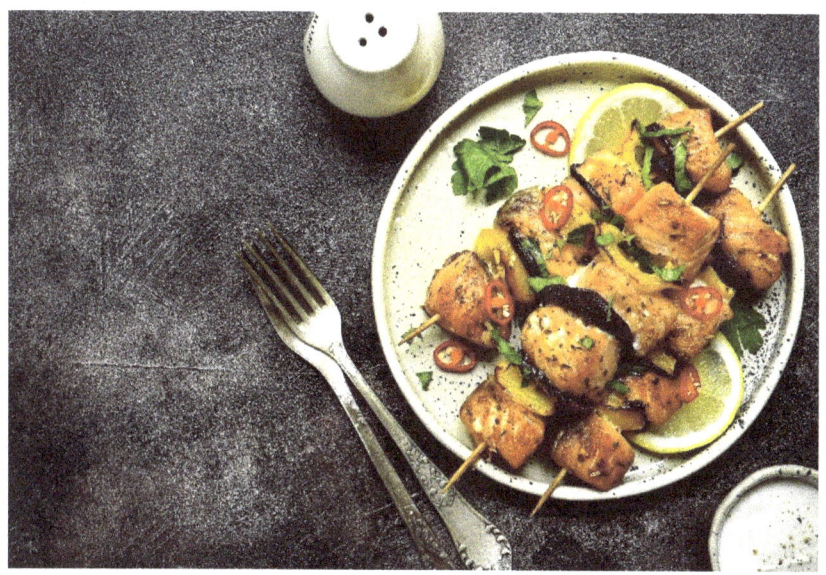

Ingredients

- 2 shallots, ends trimmed, halved
- 2 zucchinis, cut in 2-inch cubes
- 1 cup cherry tomatoes
- 6 skinless salmon fillets, cut into 1-inch pieces
- 3 limes, cut into thin wedges

Directions

1. Preheat barbecue or char grill on medium-high. Thread fish cubes onto skewers, then zucchinis, shallots and tomatoes.
2. Repeat to make 12 kebabs. Bake the kebabs for about 3 min each side for medium cooked.
3. Situate to a plate, wrap with foil and set aside for 5 min to rest.

Nutrition: 268 calories; 9g fat; 3g protein

Mediterranean Baked Salmon

Preparation: 35 min | Cooking: 11 min | Servings: 5

Ingredients

- 2 (6 oz) boneless salmon fillets
- 1 onion, tomato
- 1 tbsp. capers
- 1 tsp dry oregano
- 3 tbsp. Parmesan cheese

Directions

1. Set oven to 350 F. Place the salmon fillets in a baking dish, sprinkle with oregano, top with onion and tomato slices, drizzle with olive oil, and sprinkle with capers and Parmesan cheese.
2. Wrap the dish with foil and bake for 30 min.

Nutrition: 291 calories; 14g fat; 2g protein

Feta Cheese Baked in Foil

Preparation: 15 min | Cooking: 16 min | Servings: 5

Ingredients

- 14 oz. feta cheese, cut in slices
- 4 oz. butter
- 1 tbsp. paprika
- 1 tsp dried oregano

Directions

1. Cut the cheese into four medium-thick slices and place on sheets of butter lined aluminum foil.
2. Place a little bit of butter on top each feta cheese piece, sprinkle with paprika and dried oregano and wrap. Situate on a tray and bake in a prepared to 350 F oven for 15 min.

Nutrition: 279 calories; 9g fat; 2g protein

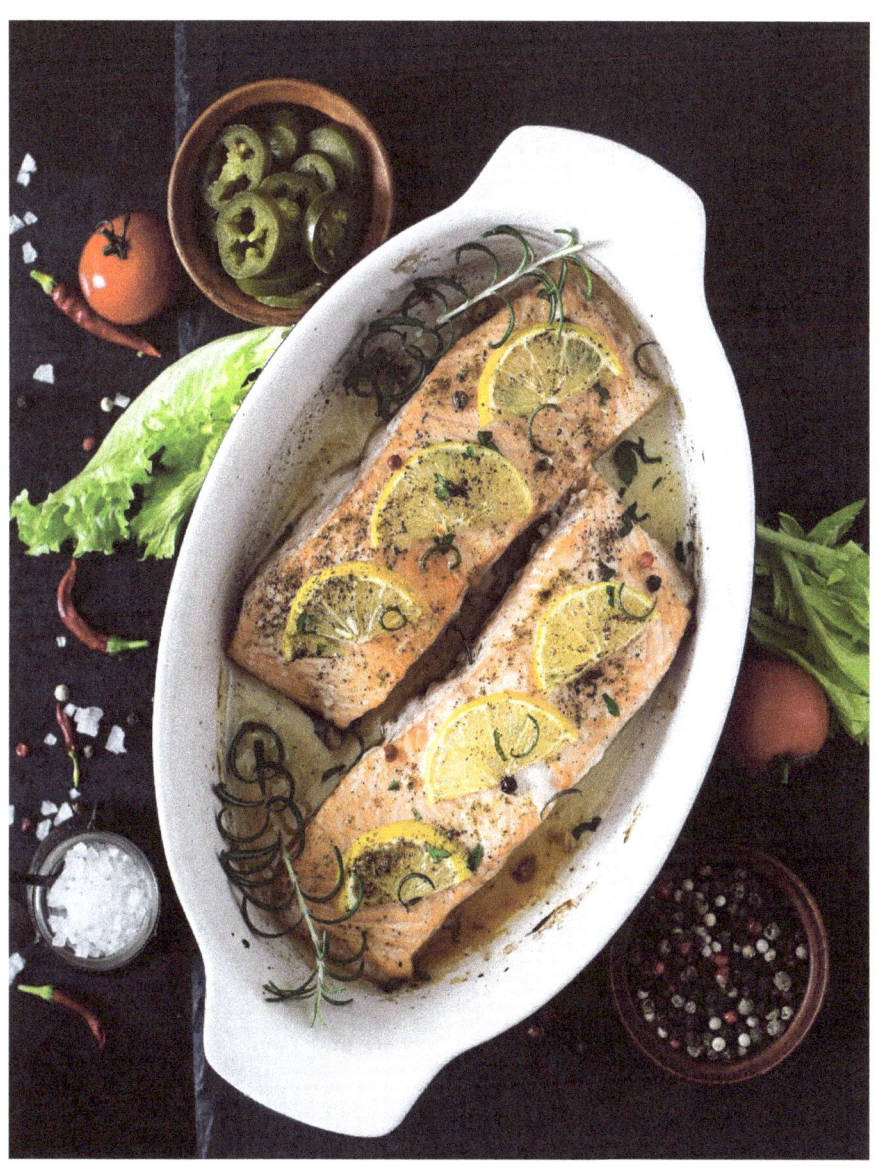

Chapter 2: Lunch & Dinner Recipes

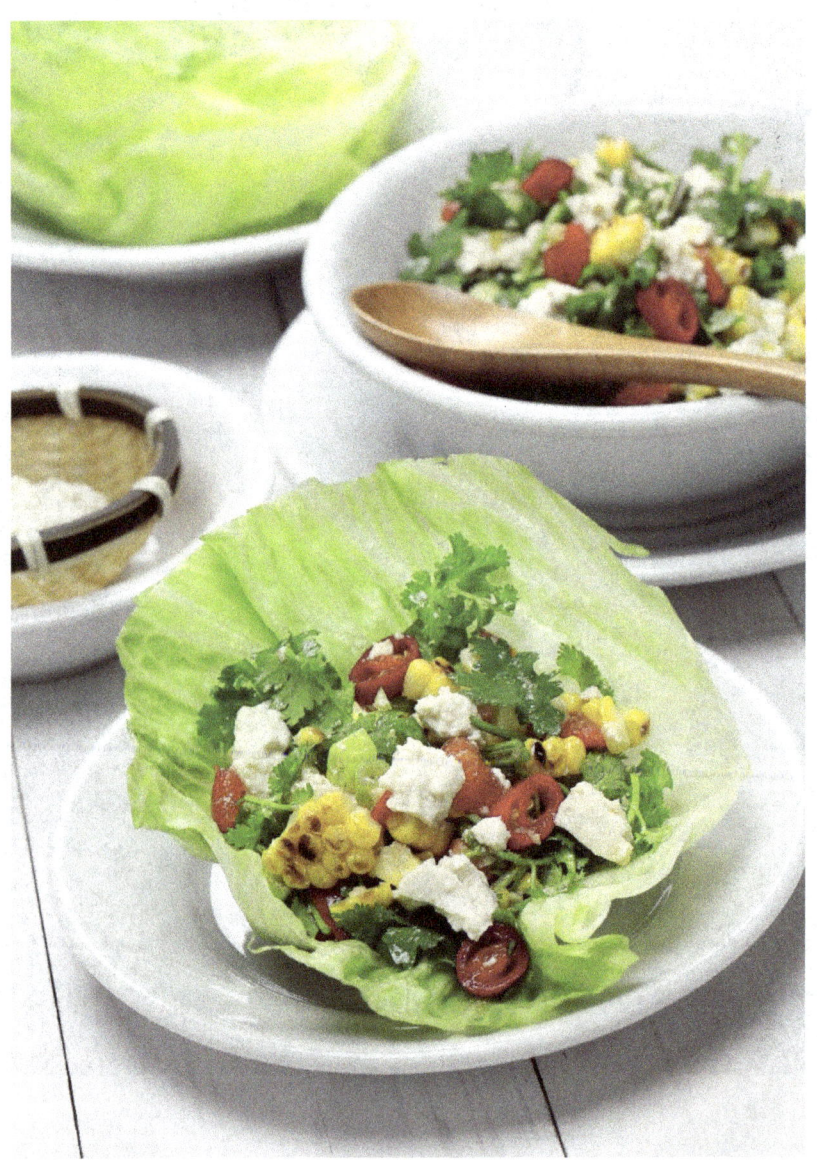

Sausage and Beans Soup

Servings: 4 | Cooking: 20 min

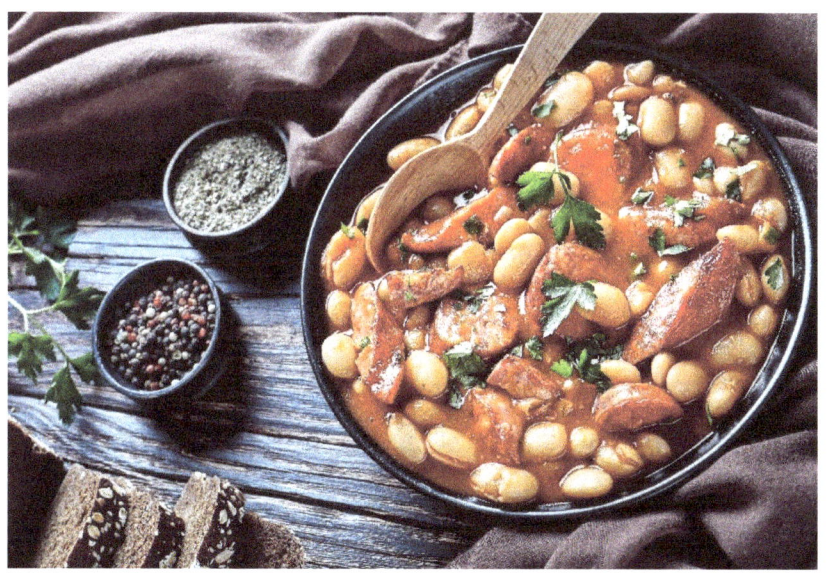

Ingredients

- 1 pound Italian pork sausage, sliced
- ¼ cup olive oil
- 1 carrot, chopped
- 1 yellow onion, chopped
- 1 celery stalk, chopped
- 2 garlic cloves, minced
- ½ pound kale, chopped
- 4 cups chicken stock

- 28 ounces canned cannellini beans, drained and rinsed
- 1 bay leaf
- 1 teaspoon rosemary, dried
- Salt and black pepper to the taste
- ½ cup parmesan, grated

Directions

1. Heat up a pot with the oil over medium heat, add the sausage and brown for 5 minutes.
2. Add the onion, carrots, garlic and celery and sauté for 3 minutes more.
3. Add the rest of the ingredients except the parmesan, bring to a simmer and cook over medium heat for 30 minutes.
4. Discard the bay leaf, ladle the soup into bowls, sprinkle the parmesan on top and serve.

Nutrition: calories 564; fat 26.5; fiber 15.4; carbs 37.4; protein 26.6

Jalapeno Grilled Salmon With Tomato Confit

Servings: 4 | Cooking: 30 min

Ingredients

- 4 salmon fillets
- 1 jalapeno
- 4 garlic cloves
- 2 tablespoons tomato paste
- 2 tablespoons olive oil
- Salt and pepper to taste
- 2 cups cherry tomatoes, halved
- 1 shallot, chopped
- 1 tablespoon olive oil

Directions

1. Combine the jalapeno, garlic, tomato paste and oil in a mortar. Mix well until a smooth paste is formed.
2. Spread the spicy paste over the salmon and season it with salt and pepper.

3. Heat a grill pan over medium flame then place the fish on the grill.
4. Cook on each side for 5-6 minutes.
5. For the confit, heat 1 tablespoon of oil in a skillet. Add the shallot and cook for 1 minute then stir in the cherry tomatoes, salt and pepper. Cook for 2 minutes on high heat.
6. Serve the grilled salmon with the tomatoes.

Nutrition: Calories:237 Fat:14.5g Protein:24.0g Carbohydrates:4.4g

Chicken And Rice Soup

Servings: 4 | Cooking: 35 min

Ingredients

- 6 cups chicken stock
- 1 and ½ cups chicken meat, cooked and shredded
- 1 bay leaf
- 1 yellow onion, chopped
- 2 tablespoons olive oil
- 1/3 cup white rice
- 1 egg, whisked
- Juice of ½ lemon
- 1 cup asparagus, trimmed and halved
- 1 cup carrots, chopped
- ½ cup dill, chopped
- Salt and black pepper to the taste

Directions

1. Heat up a pot with the oil over medium heat, add the onions and sauté for 5 minutes.

2. Add the stock, dill, the rice and the bay leaf, stir, bring to a boil over medium heat and cook for 10 minutes.
3. Add the rest of the ingredients except the egg and the lemon juice, stir and cook for 15 minutes more.
4. Add the egg whisked with the lemon juice gradually, whisk the soup, cook for 2 minutes more, divide into bowls an serve.

Nutrition: calories 263; fat 18.5; fiber 4.5; carbs 19.8; protein 14.5

Spicy Salsa Braised Beef Ribs

Servings: 12 | Cooking: 4 Hours

Ingredients

- 6 pounds beef ribs
- 4 tomatoes, diced
- 2 jalapenos, chopped
- 2 shallots, chopped
- 1 cup chopped parsley
- ½ cup chopped cilantro
- 3 tablespoons olive oil
- 2 tablespoons balsamic vinegar
- 1 teaspoon Worcestershire sauce
- Salt and pepper to taste

Directions

1. Combine the tomatoes, jalapenos, shallots, parsley, cilantro, oil, vinegar, sauce, salt and pepper in a deep dish baking pan.
2. Place the ribs in the pan and cover with aluminum foil.
3. Cook in the preheated oven at 300F for 3 1/3 hours.

4. Serve the ribs warm.

Nutrition: Calories:464 Fat:17.8g Protein:69.4g Carbohydrates:2.5g

Pork and Prunes Stew

Servings: 8 | Cooking: 1 ¼ Hours

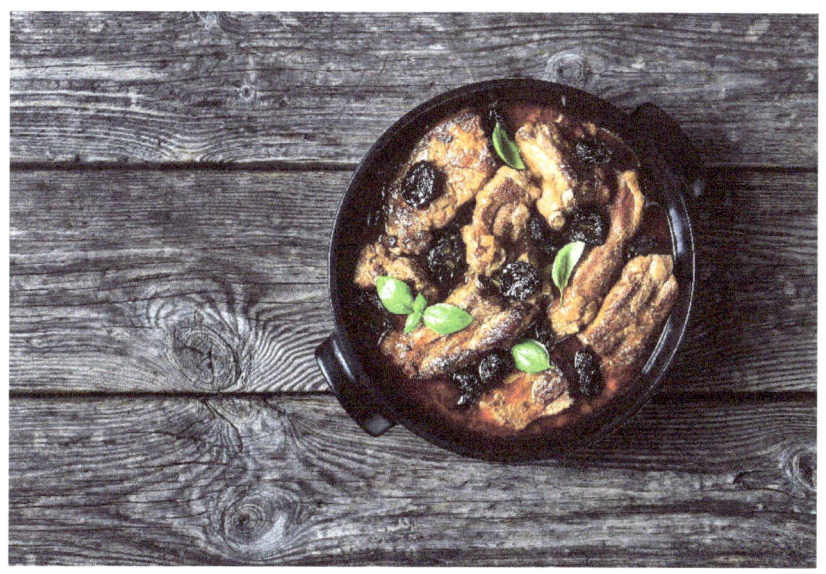

Ingredients

- 2 pounds pork tenderloin, cubed
- 2 tablespoons olive oil
- 1 sweet onions, chopped
- 4 garlic cloves, chopped
- 2 carrots, diced
- 2 celery stalks, chopped
- 2 tomatoes, peeled and diced
- 1 cup vegetable stock

- ½ cup white wine
- 1 pound prunes, pitted
- 1 bay leaf
- 1 thyme sprig
- 1 teaspoon mustard seeds
- 1 teaspoon coriander seeds
- Salt and pepper to taste

Directions

1. Combine all the ingredients in a deep dish baking pan.
2. Add salt and pepper to taste and cook in the preheated oven at 350F for 1 hour, adding more liquid as it cooks if needed.
3. Serve the stew warm and fresh.

Nutrition: Calories:363 Fat:7.9g Protein:31.7g Carbohydrates:41.4g

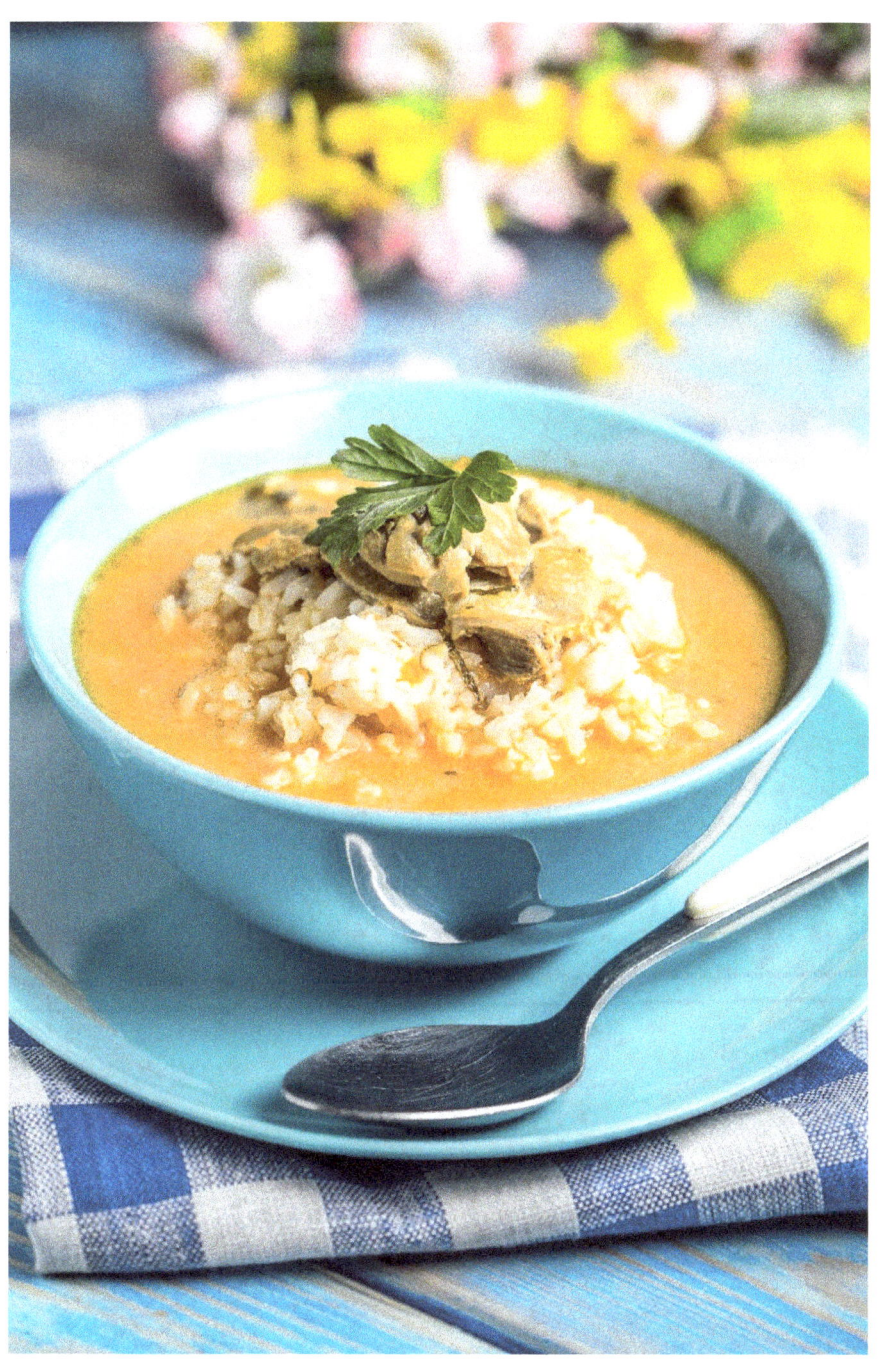

Chapter 3: Meat Recipes

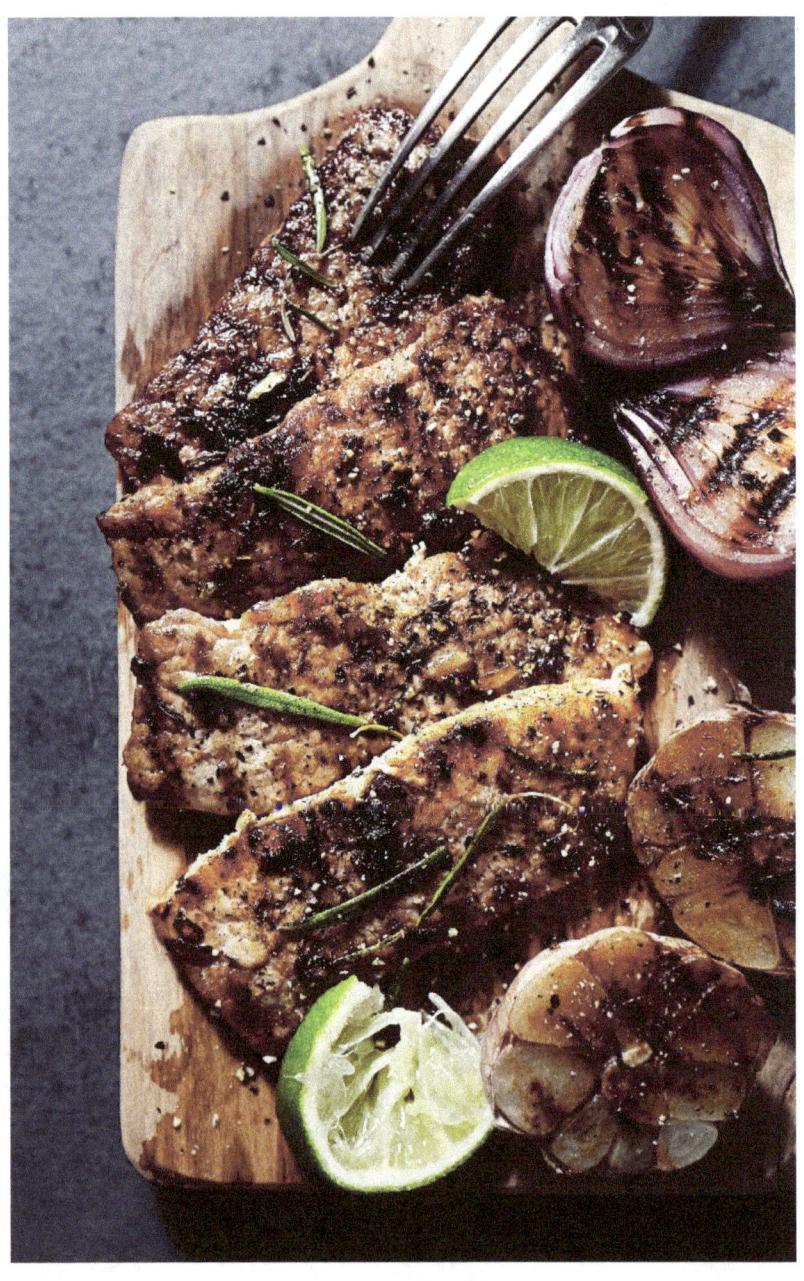

Pork And Figs Mix

Servings: 4 | Cooking: 40 min

Ingredients

- 3 tablespoons avocado oil
- 1 and ½ pounds pork stew meat, roughly cubed
- Salt and black pepper to the taste
- 1 cup red onions, chopped
- 1 cup figs, dried and chopped
- 1 tablespoon ginger, grated
- 1 tablespoon garlic, minced
- 1 cup canned tomatoes, crushed
- 2 tablespoons parsley, chopped

Directions

1. Heat up a pot with the oil over medium-high heat, add the meat and brown for 5 minutes.
2. Add the onions and sauté for 5 minutes more.
3. Add the rest of the ingredients, bring to a simmer and cook over medium heat for 30 minutes more.
4. Divide the mix between plates and serve.

Nutrition: calories 309; fat 16; fiber 10.4; carbs 21.1; protein 34.2

Lamb Chops

Servings: 1 Chop | Cooking: 6 min

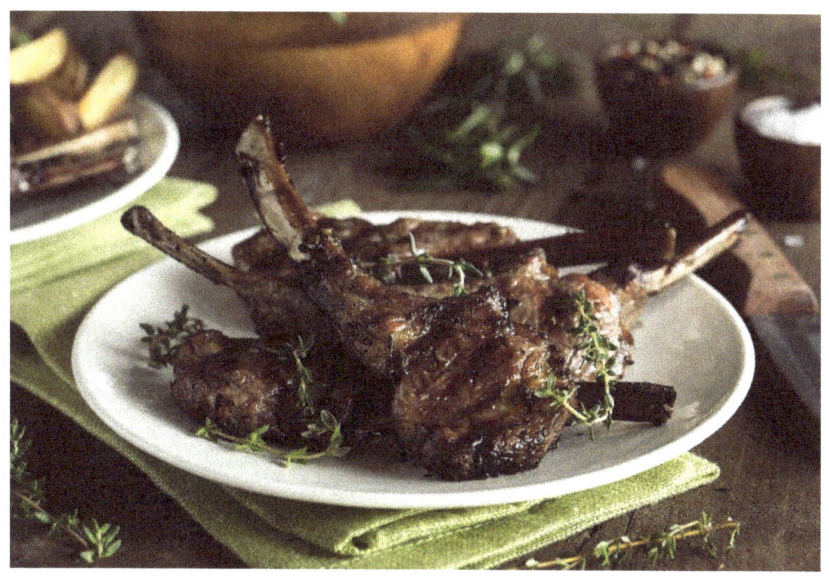

Ingredients

- 6 (3/4-in.-thick) lamb chops
- 2 TB. fresh rosemary, finely chopped
- 3 TB. minced garlic
- 1 tsp. salt
- 1 tsp. ground black pepper
- 3 TB. extra-virgin olive oil

Directions

1. In a large bowl, combine lamb chops, rosemary, garlic, salt, black pepper, and extra-virgin olive oil until chops are evenly coated. Let chops marinate at room temperature for at least 25 minutes.
2. Preheat a grill to medium heat.
3. Place chops on the grill, and cook for 3 minutes per side for medium well.
4. Serve warm.

Chicken Quinoa Pilaf

Servings: 1 Cup | Cooking: 35 min

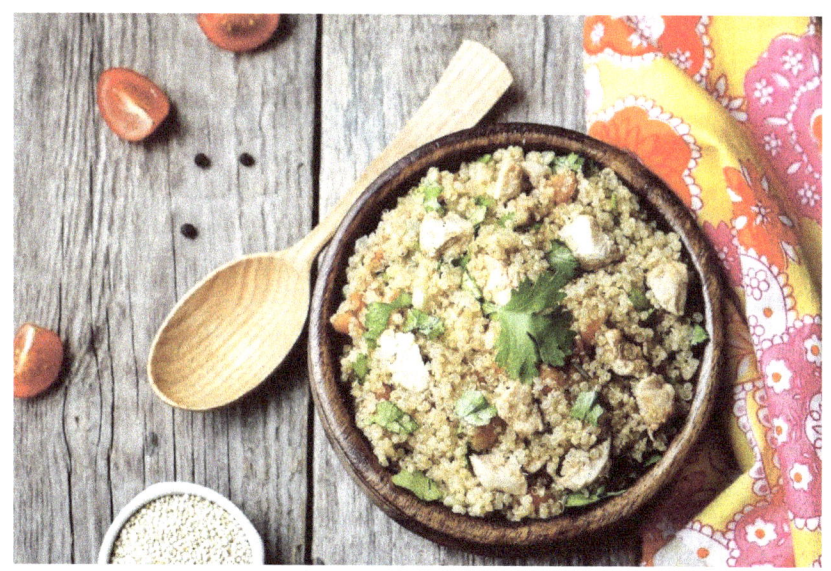

Ingredients

- 2 (8-oz.) boneless, skinless chicken breasts, cut into 1/2-in. cubes
- 3 TB. extra-virgin olive oil
- 1 medium red onion, finely chopped
- 1 TB. minced garlic
- 1 (16-oz.) can diced tomatoes, with juice
- 2 cups water
- 2 tsp. salt

- 1 TB. dried oregano
- 1 TB. turmeric
- 1 tsp. paprika
- 1 tsp. ground black pepper
- 2 cups red or yellow quinoa
- 1/2 cup fresh parsley, chopped

Directions

1. In a large, 3-quart pot over medium heat, heat extra-virgin olive oil. Add chicken, and cook for 5 minutes.
2. Add red onion and garlic, stir, and cook for 5 minutes.
3. Add tomatoes with juice, water, salt, oregano, turmeric, paprika, and black pepper. Stir, and simmer for 5 minutes.
4. Add red quinoa, and stir. Cover, reduce heat to low, and cook for 20 minutes. Remove from heat.
5. Fluff with a fork, cover again, and let sit for 10 minutes.
6. Serve warm.

Greek Styled Lamb Chops

Servings: 4 | Cooking: 4 min

Ingredients

- ¼ tsp black pepper
- ½ tsp salt
- 1 tbsp bottled minced garlic
- 1 tbsp dried oregano
- 2 tbsp lemon juice
- 8 pcs of lamb loin chops, around 4 oz
- Cooking: spray

Directions

1. Preheat broiler.
2. In a big bowl or dish, combine the black pepper, salt, minced garlic, lemon juice and oregano. Then rub it equally on all sides of the lamb chops.
3. Then coat a broiler pan with the cooking spray before placing the lamb chops on the pan and broiling until desired doneness is reached or for four minutes.

Nutrition: Calories: 131.9; Carbs: 2.6g; Protein: 17.1g; Fat: 5.9g

Bulgur And Chicken Skillet

Servings: 4 | Cooking: 40 min

Ingredients

- 4 (6-oz.) skinless, boneless chicken breasts
- 1 tablespoon olive oil, divided
- 1 cup thinly sliced red onion
- 1 tablespoon thinly sliced garlic
- 1 cup unsalted chicken stock
- 1 tablespoon coarsely chopped fresh dill
- 1/2 teaspoon freshly ground black pepper, divided
- 1/2 cup uncooked bulgur
- 2 teaspoons chopped fresh or 1/2 tsp. dried oregano
- 4 cups chopped fresh kale (about 2 1/2 oz.)
- 1/2 cup thinly sliced bottled roasted red bell peppers
- 2 ounces feta cheese, crumbled (about 1/2 cup)
- 3/4 teaspoon kosher salt, divided

Directions

1. Place a cast iron skillet on medium high fire and heat for 5 minutes. Add oil and heat for 2 minutes.

2. Season chicken with pepper and salt to taste.
3. Brown chicken for 4 minutes per side and transfer to a plate.
4. In same skillet, sauté garlic and onion for 3 minutes. Stir in oregano and bulgur and toast for 2 minutes.
5. Stir in kale and bell pepper, cook for 2 minutes. Pour in stock and season well with pepper and salt.
6. Return chicken to skillet and turn off fire. Pop in a preheated 400oF oven and bake for 15 minutes.
7. Remove form oven, fluff bulgur and turn over chicken. Let it stand for 5 minutes.
8. Serve and enjoy with a sprinkle of feta cheese.

Nutrition: Calories: 369; Carbs: 21.0g; Protein: 45.0g; Fats: 11.3g

Chapter 4: Poultry Recipes

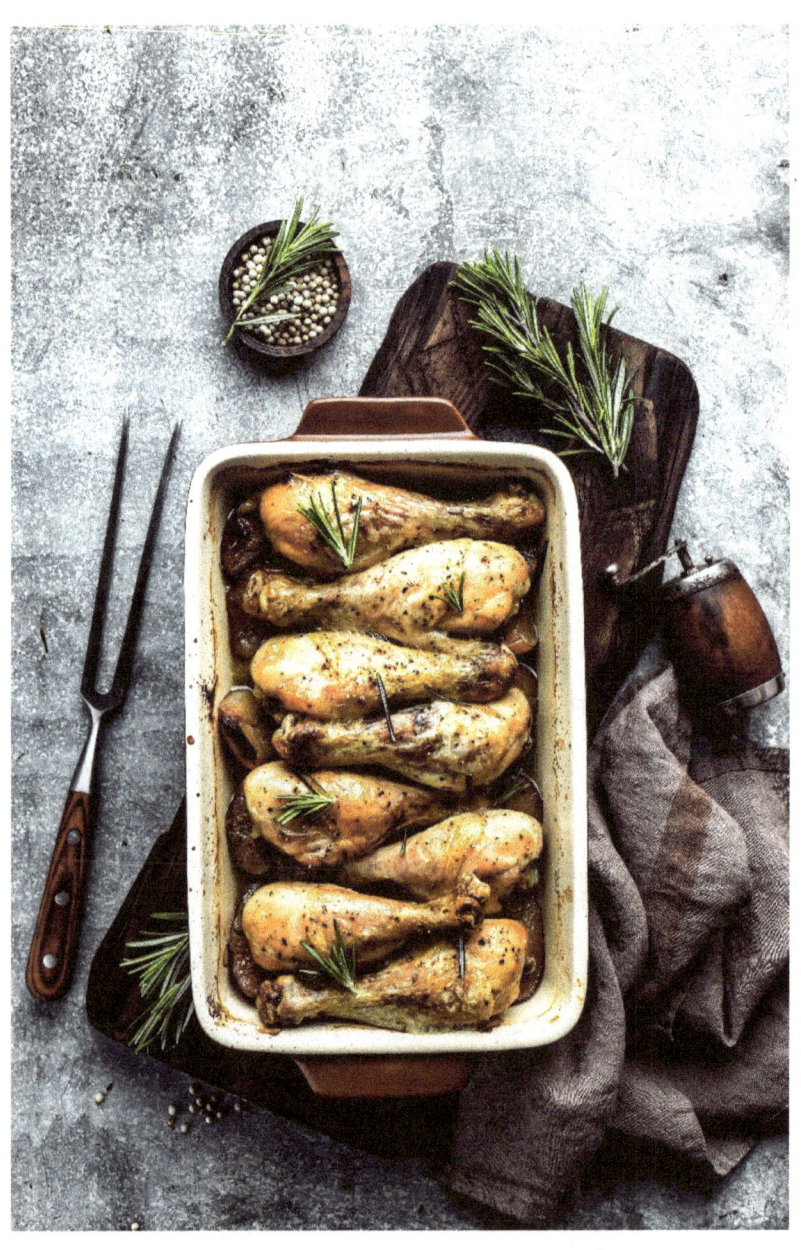

Chicken And Spinach Cakes

Servings: 4 | Cooking: 15 min

Ingredients
- 8 oz ground chicken
- 1 cup fresh spinach, blended
- 1 teaspoon minced onion
- ½ teaspoon salt
- 1 red bell pepper, grinded
- 1 egg, beaten
- 1 teaspoon ground black pepper
- 4 tablespoons Panko breadcrumbs

Directions
1. In the mixing bowl mix up together ground chicken, blended spinach, minced garlic, salt, grinded bell pepper, egg, and ground black pepper.
2. When the chicken mixture is smooth, make 4 burgers from it and coat them in Panko breadcrumbs.
3. Place the burgers in the non-sticky baking dish or line the baking tray with baking paper.
4. Bake the burgers for 15 minutes at 365F.

5. Flip the chicken burgers on another side after 7 minutes of cooking.

Nutrition: calories 171; fat 5.7; fiber 1.7; carbs 10.5; protein 19.4

Cream Cheese Chicken

Servings: 2 | Cooking: 20 min

Ingredients

- 1 onion, chopped
- 1 sweet red pepper, roasted, chopped
- 1 cup spinach, chopped
- ½ cup cream
- 1 teaspoon cream cheese
- 1 tablespoon olive oil
- ½ teaspoon ground black pepper
- 8 oz chicken breast, skinless, boneless, sliced

Directions

1. Mix up together sliced chicken breast with ground black pepper and put in the saucepan.
2. Add olive oil and mix up.
3. Roast the chicken for 5 minutes over the medium-high heat. Stir it from time to time.
4. After this, add chopped sweet pepper, onion, and cream cheese.
5. Mix up well and bring to boil.
6. Add spinach and cream. Mix up well.

7. Close the lid and cook chicken Alfredo for 10 minutes more over the medium heat.

Nutrition: calories 279; fat 14; fiber 2.5; carbs 12.4; protein 26.4

Chicken And Lemongrass Sauce

Servings: 4 | Cooking: 20 min

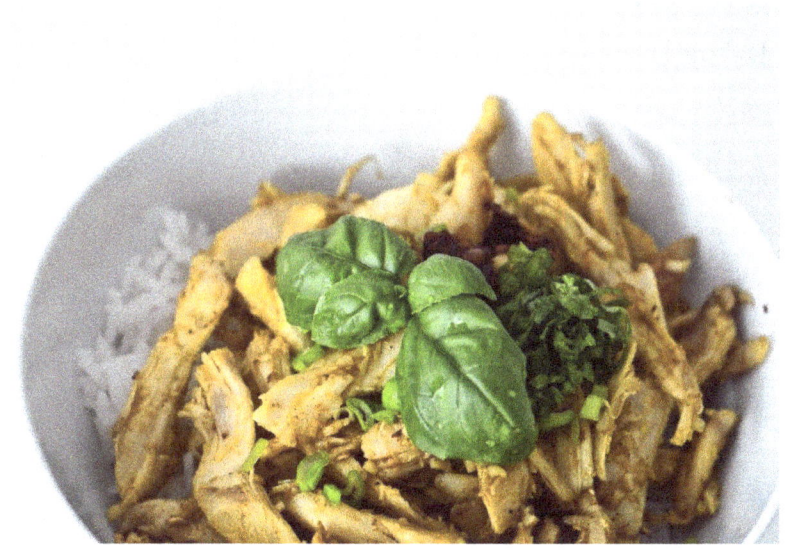

Ingredients

- 1 tablespoon dried dill
- 1 teaspoon butter, melted
- ½ teaspoon lemongrass
- ½ teaspoon cayenne pepper
- 1 teaspoon tomato sauce
- 3 tablespoons sour cream
- 1 teaspoon salt
- 10 oz chicken fillet, cubed

Directions

1. Make the sauce: in the saucepan whisk together lemongrass, tomato sauce, sour cream, salt, and dried dill.
2. Bring the sauce to boil.
3. Meanwhile, pour melted butter in the skillet.
4. Add cubed chicken fillet and roast it for 5 minutes. Stir it from time to time.
5. Then place the chicken cubes in the hot sauce.
6. Close the lid and cook the meal for 10 minutes over the low heat.

Nutrition: calories 166; fat 8.2; fiber 0.2; carbs 1.1; protein 21

Spiced Chicken Meatballs

Servings: 4 | Cooking: 20 min

Ingredients
- 1 pound chicken meat, ground
- 1 tablespoon pine nuts, toasted and chopped
- 1 egg, whisked
- 2 teaspoons turmeric powder
- 2 garlic cloves, minced
- Salt and black pepper to the taste
- 1 and ¼ cups heavy cream
- 2 tablespoons olive oil
- ¼ cup parsley, chopped
- 1 tablespoon chives, chopped

Directions
1. In a bowl, combine the chicken with the pine nuts and the rest of the ingredients except the oil and the cream, stir well and shape medium meatballs out of this mix.
2. Heat up a pan with the oil over medium-high heat, add the meatballs and cook them for 4 minutes on each side.

3. Add the cream, toss gently, cook everything over medium heat for 10 minutes more, divide between plates and serve.

Nutrition: calories 283; fat 9.2; fiber 12.8; carbs 24.4; protein 34.5

Paprika Chicken Wings

Servings: 4 | Cooking: 8 min

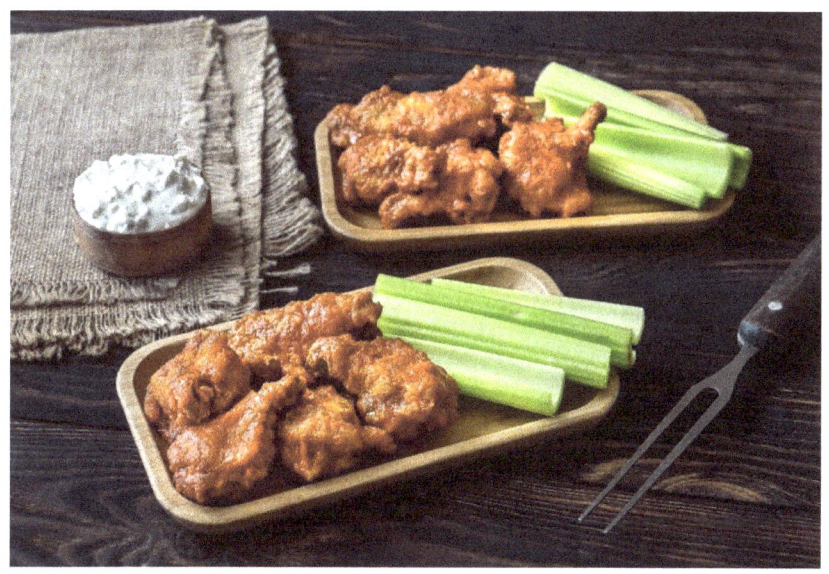

Ingredients:

- 4 chicken wings, boneless
- 1 tablespoon honey
- ½ teaspoon paprika
- ¼ teaspoon cayenne pepper
- ¾ teaspoon ground black pepper
- 1 tablespoon lemon juice
- ½ teaspoon sunflower oil

Directions

1. Make the honey marinade: whisk together honey, paprika, cayenne pepper, ground black pepper, lemon juice, and sunflower oil.
2. Then brush the chicken wings with marinade carefully.
3. Preheat the grill to 385F.
4. Place the chicken wings in the grill and cook them for 4 minutes from each side.

Nutrition: calories 26; fat 0.8; fiber 0.3; carbs 5.1; protein 0.3

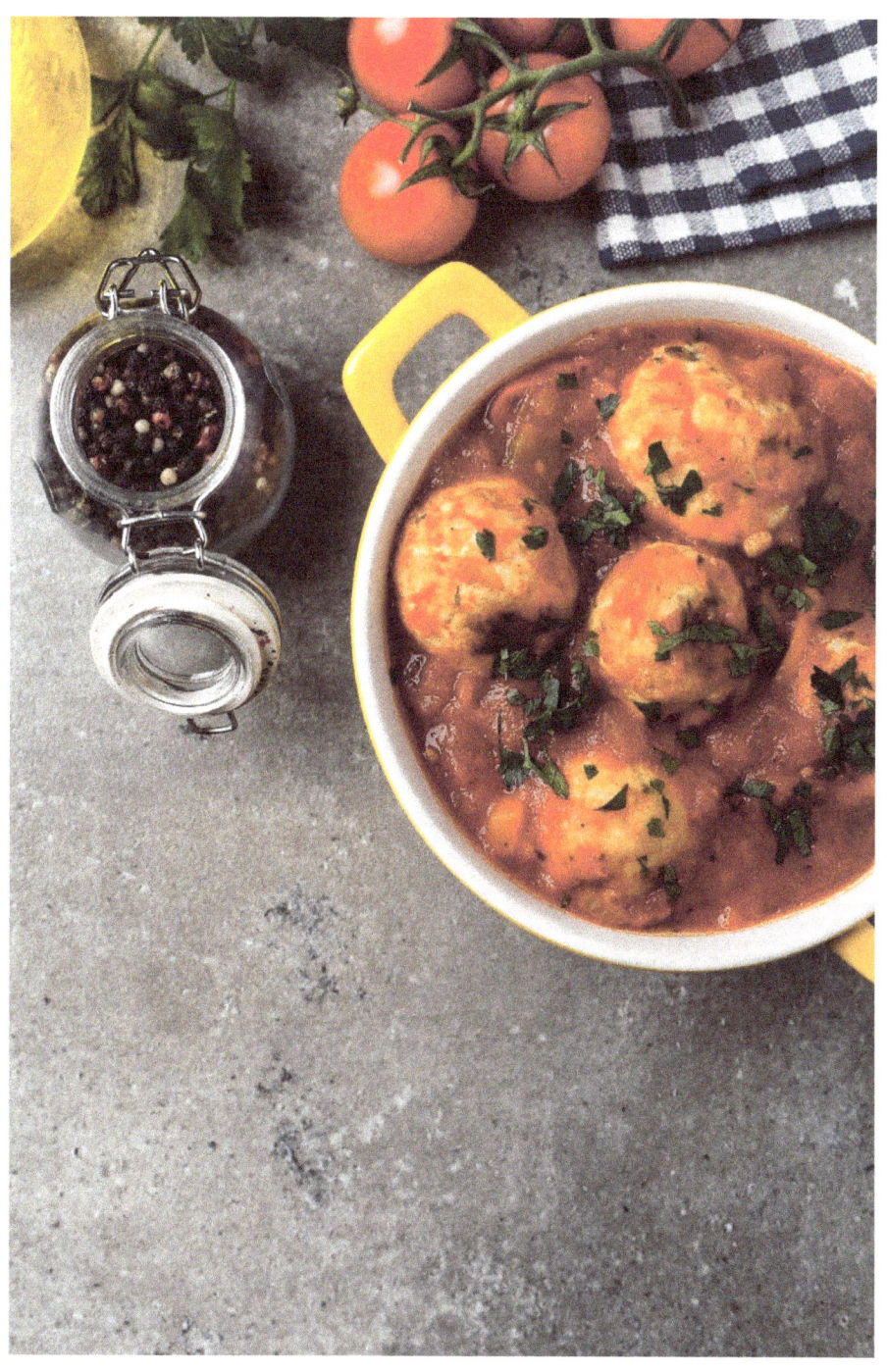

Chapter 5: Fish and Seafood Recipes

Fried Salmon

Servings: 2 | Cooking: 8 min

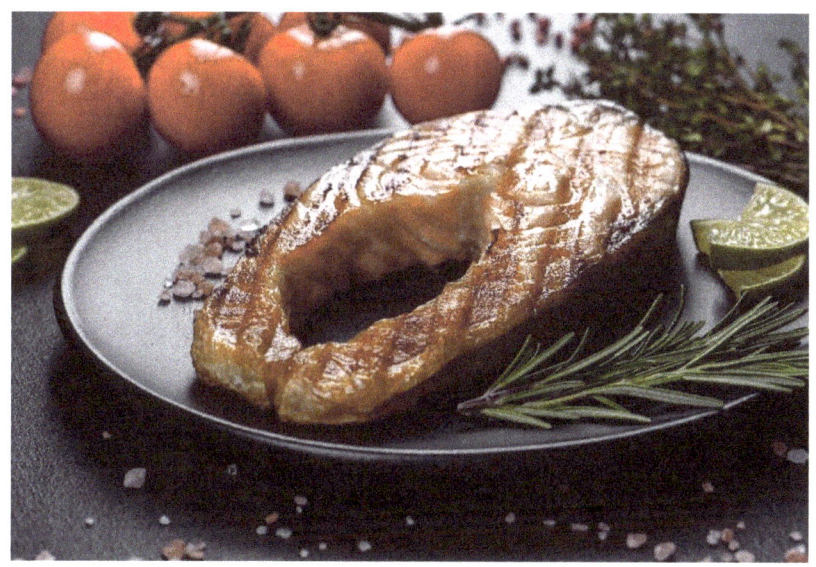

Ingredients

- 5 oz salmon fillet
- ¼ teaspoon salt
- ½ teaspoon ground black pepper
- 1 tablespoon sunflower oil
- ¼ teaspoon lime juice

Directions

1. Cut the salmon fillet on 2 lengthwise pieces.

2. Sprinkle every fish piece with salt, ground black pepper, and lime juice.
3. Pour sunflower oil in the skillet and preheat it until shimmering.
4. Then place fish fillets in the hot oil and cook them for 3 minutes from each side.

Nutrition: calories 157; fat 11.4; fiber 0.1; carbs 0.3; protein 13.8

Smoked Salmon And Veggies Mix

Servings: 4 | Cooking: 20 min

Ingredients

- 3 red onions, cut into wedges
- ¾ cup green olives, pitted and halved
- 3 red bell peppers, roughly chopped
- ½ teaspoon smoked paprika
- Salt and black pepper to the taste
- 3 tablespoons olive oil
- 4 salmon fillets, skinless and boneless
- 2 tablespoons chives, chopped

Directions

1. In a roasting pan, combine the salmon with the onions and the rest of the ingredients, introduce in the oven and bake at 390 degrees F for 20 minutes.
2. Divide the mix between plates and serve.

Nutrition: calories 301; fat 5.9; fiber 11.9; carbs 26.4; protein 22.4

Berries And Grilled Calamari

Servings: 4 | Cooking: 5 min

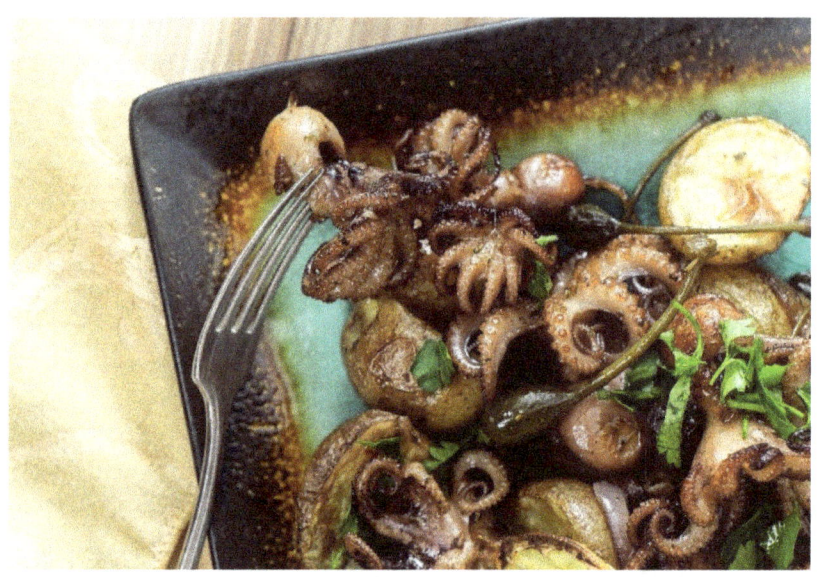

Ingredients

- ¼ cup dried cranberries
- ¼ cup extra virgin olive oil
- ¼ cup olive oil
- ¼ cup sliced almonds
- ½ lemon, juiced
- ¾ cup blueberries
- 1 ½ pounds calamari tube, cleaned
- 1 granny smith apple, sliced thinly

- 1 tablespoon fresh lemon juice
- 2 tablespoons apple cider vinegar
- 6 cups fresh spinach
- Freshly grated pepper to taste
- Sea salt to taste

Directions

1. In a small bowl, make the vinaigrette by mixing well the tablespoon of lemon juice, apple cider vinegar, and extra virgin olive oil. Season with pepper and salt to taste. Set aside.
2. Turn on the grill to medium fire and let the grates heat up for a minute or two.
3. In a large bowl, add olive oil and the calamari tube. Season calamari generously with pepper and salt.
4. Place seasoned and oiled calamari onto heated grate and grill until cooked or opaque. This is around two minutes per side.
5. As you wait for the calamari to cook, you can combine almonds, cranberries, blueberries, spinach, and the thinly sliced apple in a large salad bowl. Toss to mix.

6. Remove cooked calamari from grill and transfer on a chopping board. Cut into ¼-inch thick rings and throw into the salad bowl.
7. Drizzle with vinaigrette and toss well to coat salad.
8. Serve and enjoy!

Nutrition: Calories: 567; Fat: 24.5g; Protein: 54.8g; Carbs: 30.6g

Salmon And Zucchini Rolls

Servings: 8 | Cooking: 0 min

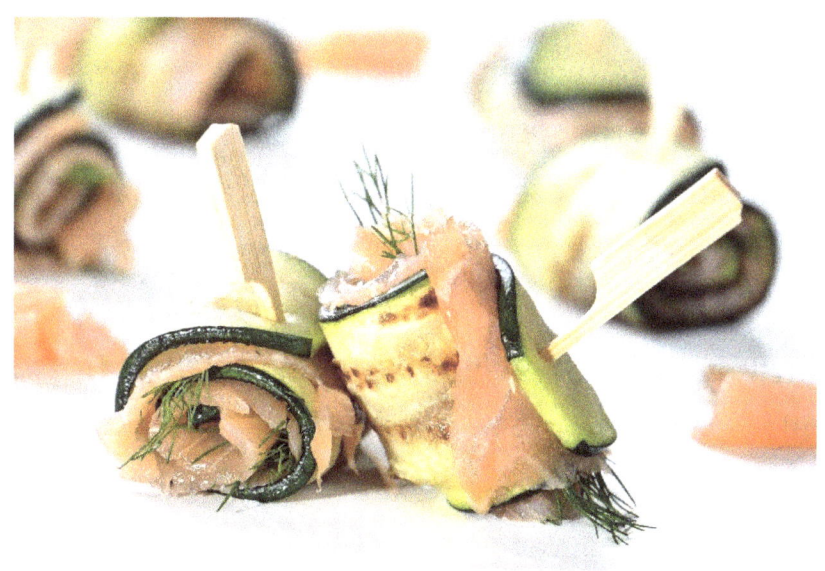

Ingredients

- 8 slices smoked salmon, boneless
- 2 zucchinis, sliced lengthwise in 8 pieces
- 1 cup ricotta cheese, soft
- 2 teaspoons lemon zest, grated
- 1 tablespoon dill, chopped
- 1 small red onion, sliced
- Salt and pepper to the taste

Directions

1. In a bowl, mix the ricotta cheese with the rest of the ingredients except the salmon and the zucchini and whisk well.
2. Arrange the zucchini slices on a working surface, and divide the salmon on top.
3. Spread the cheese mix all over, roll and secure with toothpicks and serve right away.

Nutrition: calories 297; fat 24.3; fiber 11.6; carbs 15.4; protein 11.6

Scallions And Salmon Tartar

Servings: 4 | Cooking: 0 min

Ingredients

- 4 tablespoons scallions, chopped
- 2 teaspoons lemon juice
- 1 tablespoon chives, minced
- 1 tablespoon olive oil
- 1 pound salmon, skinless, boneless and minced
- Salt and black pepper to the taste
- 1 tablespoon parsley, chopped

Directions

1. In a bowl, combine the scallions with the salmon and the rest of the ingredients, stir well, divide into small molds between plates and serve.

Nutrition: calories 224; fat 14.5; fiber 5.2; carbs 12.7; protein 5.3

Chapter 6: Salads & Side Dishes

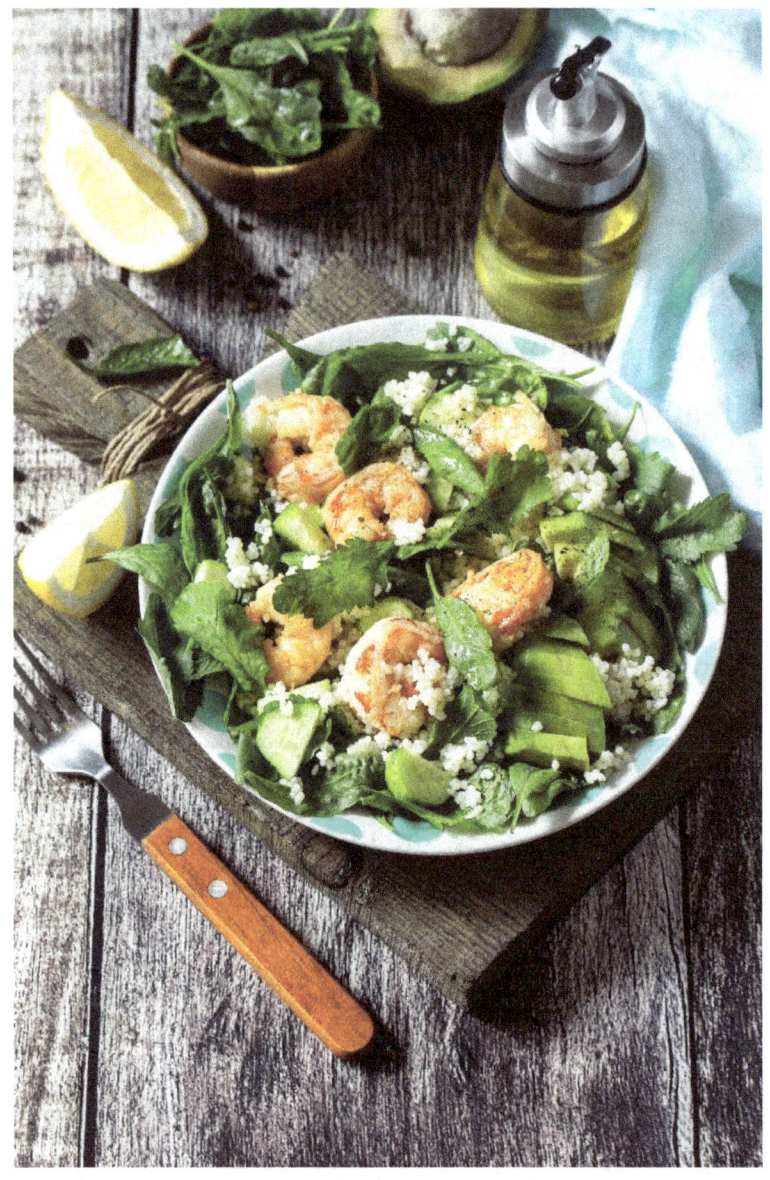

Instant Pot Collard Greens with Tomatoes

Preparation: 18 min | Cooking: 8 min | Servings: 4

Ingredients

- 1 white onion (diced)
- 3tbsp olive oil
- 3 garlic cloves (minced)
- Cup tomatoes (sun-dried and chopped)
- 1 bunch collard greens (roughly cut and hard stems removed)

Directions

1. Turn on the sauté function on your instant pot.
2. Add onions and olive oil to the instant pot and let cook for three min or lightly browned.
3. Mix in the rest of ingredients simultaneously while stirring.
4. Add salt and pepper to taste and a cup of water. Turn off the sauté function and set to manual. Set time for five min at high pressure.
5. When the time has elapsed, release pressure naturally.

6. Open the lid and drizzle a half lemon juice.
7. Serve and enjoy.

Nutrition: 498 Calories: 19g Protein: 32g Carbohydrates

Instant Pot Millet Pilaf

Preparation: 23 min | Cooking: 11 min | Servings: 4

Ingredients

- 1 cup millet
- Cup apricot and shelled pistachios (roughly chopped)
- 1 lemon juice and zest
- 1 tbsp. olive oil
- Cup parsley (fresh)

Directions

1. Pour one and three-quarter cup of water in your instant pot. Place the millet and lid the instant pot.
2. Adjust time for 10 min on high pressure. When the time has elapsed, release pressure naturally.
3. Remove the lid and add all other ingredients. Stir while adjusting the seasonings.
4. Serve and enjoy

Nutrition: 308 Calories: 11g Fat 6g Fiber

Barley & Mushroom Soup

Preparation: 7 min | Cooking: 27 min | Servings: 6

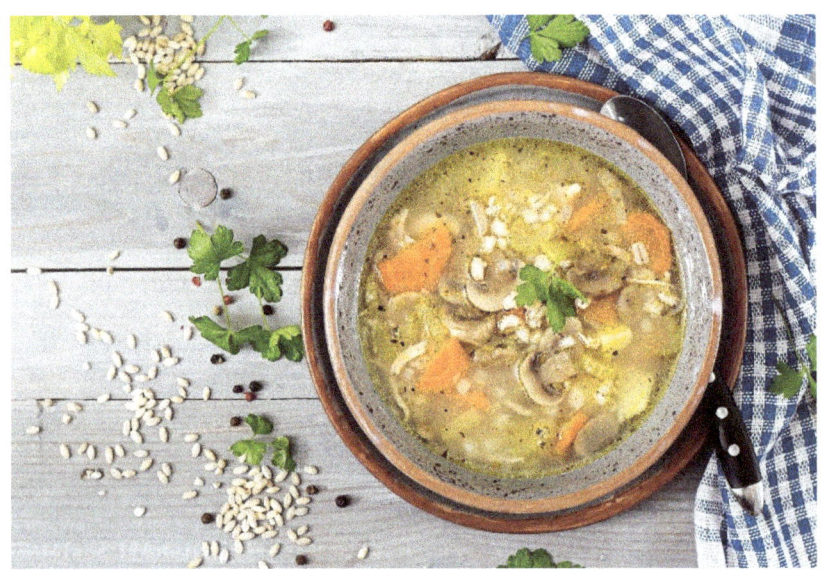

Ingredients

- ¼ cup red wine
- 2 tablespoons olive oil
- 1 cup carrots, chopped
- 1 cup onion, chopped
- ½ cups mushrooms, chopped
- 2 cups vegetable broth, low sodium
- 1 cup pearled barley, uncooked
- 2 tablespoons tomato paste

- 1 bay leaf
- 6 tablespoons parmesan cheese, grated
- 4 sprigs thyme, fresh

Directions

1. Get out a stockpot and place it over medium heat. Heat your oil and add in your carrots and onion. Cook for five min and frequently stir during this time.
2. Turn your heat up to medium-high before throwing in your mushrooms. Cook for another three min. Make sure to stir frequently.
3. Add in your barley, tomato paste, thyme, wine, broth, and bay leaf. Stir and cover. Bring to boil, and stir a few more times. Reduce to medium-low heat. Cover, and cook for another twelve to fifteen min.
4. Remove your bay leaf and serve topped with cheese.

Nutrition: Calories: 491; Fat: 12g; Protein: 19g

Instant Pot Stuffed Sweet Potatoes

Preparation: 13 min | Cooking: 22 min | Servings: 2

Ingredients

- 2 sweet potatoes (washed thoroughly)
- cup chickpeas, onions
- 2 spring onions
- 1 avocado
- cooked couscous

Directions

1. Pour a cup and half of water in your instant pot then place steam rack in place.
2. Place the sweet potatoes on the rack. Set the valve to sealing and time for seventeen min under high pressure.
3. Meanwhile, roast the chickpeas on your pan with olive oil.
4. Add salt and pepper to taste then paprika. Stir until chickpeas are coated evenly.
5. Cook for a minute then put off the heat.
6. When the instant pot time elapses, release pressure naturally for five min. Let the sweet

potatoes cool then remove them from the instant pot.
7. Cut the sweet potatoes lengthwise and use a fork to mash the inside creating a space for toppings.
8. Add the pre-prepared toppings then serve with feta cheese lemon wedges.

Nutrition: 776 Calories; 26g Fat; 23g Protein;

Instant Pot Couscous and Vegetable Medley

Preparation: 9 min | Cooking: 17 min | Servings: 3

Ingredients
- Onion (chopped)
- 1 red bell pepper (chopped)
- cup couscous Israeli, carrot
- Garam masala, cilantro, lemon juice,
- 2 bays leave

Directions
1. Put on sauté function on your instant pot then add olive oil.
2. Add bay leaves followed by chopped onions the sauté for two min.
3. Add pepper and carrots then continue to sauté for one more minute.
4. Stir in couscous, Garam masala, salt to taste and a cup and three-quarter of water.
5. Switch the sauté function to manual and set for two min. When the time has elapsed naturally release pressure for ten min.

6. Fluff the couscous then mix in lemon juice and garnish with cilantro.
7. Remove from instant pot and serve when hot

Nutrition: 460 Calories: 5g Fat 13g Protein

Chickpea Pasta Salad

Preparation: 8 min | Cooking: 17 min | Servings: 6

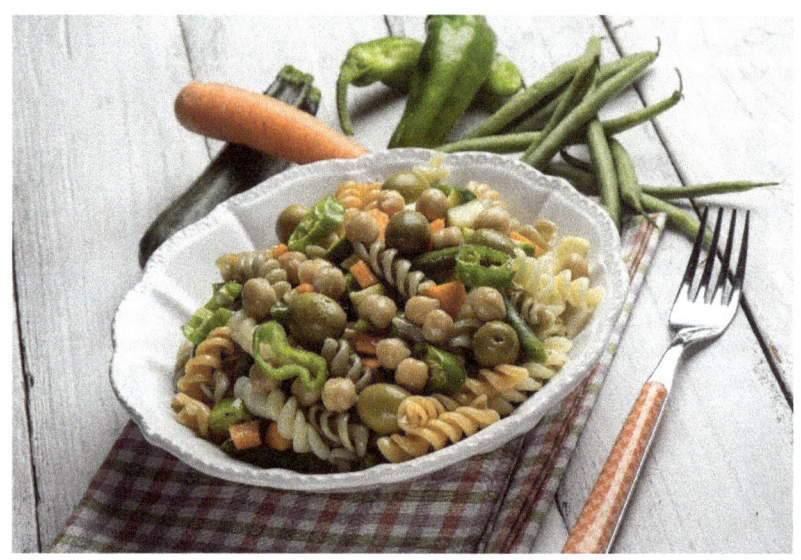

Ingredients

- 2 tablespoons olive oil
- 16 ounces rotelle pasta
- ½ cup cured olives, chopped
- 2 tablespoons oregano, fresh & minced
- 2 tablespoons parsley, fresh & chopped
- 1 bunch green onions, chopped
- ¼ cup red wine vinegar

- 15 ounces canned garbanzo beans, drained & rinsed
- ½ cup parmesan cheese, grated
- sea salt & black pepper to taste

Directions

1. Bring water to boil and cook your pasta al dente per package instructions. Drain it and rinse it using cold water.
2. Get out a skillet and heat your olive oil over medium heat. Add in your scallions, chickpeas, parsley, oregano, and olives. Set the heat to low then cook for twenty min more. Allow this mixture to cool.
3. Toss your chickpea mixture with your pasta and add in your grated cheese, salt, pepper, and vinegar. Chill before serving.

Nutrition: Calories: 445; Fat: 9g; Protein: 13g

Bean Lettuce Wraps

Preparation: 9 min | Cooking: 7 min | Servings: 4

Ingredients

- 15 ounces cannellini beans, canned, drained & rinsed sea salt & black pepper to taste
- ¾ cup tomatoes, fresh & chopped
- ½ cup red onion, diced
- 1 tbsp. olive oil
- ¼ cup parsley, fresh & chopped fine
- 8 romaine lettuce leaves
- ½ cup hummus

Directions

1. Get out a skillet and place it over medium heat. Heat your oil. Once your oil is hot, adding in your onion, and cook for three min. Stir occasionally.
2. Stir in your tomatoes and season with salt and pepper. Cook for another three min. Add in your beans and heat all the way through. Stir it, so it doesn't burn. Remove it from heat, and then mix in your parsley.

3. Spread a tablespoon of hummus on each lettuce leaf and then top with your bean mixture. Fold, and then wrap before serving.

Nutrition: Calories: 405; Fat: 6g; Protein: 10g

Easy Lentil & Rice Bowl

Preparation: 6 min | Cooking: 29 min | Servings: 4

Ingredients

- ¼ cup parsley, curly leaf, fresh & chopped
- 1 ½ tablespoons olive oil
- sea salt & black pepper to taste
- 1 clove garlic, minced
- 1 tablespoon lemon juice, fresh
- 1 (6-oz.) can onion, drained
- ½ cup celery, diced
- ½ cup carrots, diced
- ½ cup instant brown rice, uncooked
- ½ cup green lentils, uncooked
- ¼ vegetable broth, low sodium

Directions

1. Put a saucepan over high heat, and then bring your lentils to a boil with the broth. Cover once it begins to boil, and then lower the heat to medium-low. Cook for eight min.

2. Set the heat to medium, and add in your rice. Stir well, and cover. Cook for fifteen more min. The liquid should be absorbed.
3. Allow it to set off the heat and cover for one minute before stirring.
4. Mix your celery, olives, onion, carrot, and parsley in a bowl while your rice and lentils are cooking.
5. Get out a bowl and whisk your oil, lemon juice, salt, pepper, and garlic together. Set this to the side.
6. When your rice and lentils are cooked, add them to a serving bowl and top with the dressing. Serve immediately.

Nutrition: Calories: 391; Fat: 8g; Protein: 12g

Chickpea Pita Patties

Preparation: 12 min | Cooking: 21 min | Servings: 4

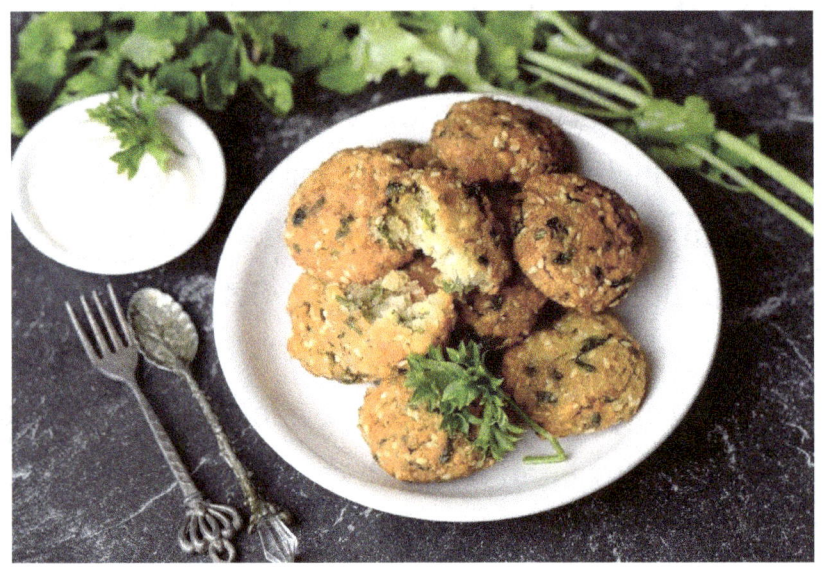

Ingredients

- egg, large
- teaspoons oregano
- ½ cup panko bread crumbs, whole wheat sea salt & black pepper to taste
- 1 tablespoon olive oil
- 1 cucumber, halved lengthwise 6 ounces Greek yogurt, 2%
- clove garlic, minced

- pita bread, whole wheat & halved
- 1 tomato, cut into 4 thick slices
- ½ cup hummus
- 15 ounces chickpeas, drained & rinsed

Directions

1. Get out a large bowl, mash your chickpeas with a potato masher, and then add in your bread crumbs, eggs, hummus, oregano, and pepper. Stir well. Form four patties, and then press them flat on a plate. They should be ¾ inch thick.
2. Get out a skillet, placing it over medium-high heat. Heat the oil until hot, which should take three min. Cook the patties for five min per side.
3. While your patties are cooking, shred half of your cucumber with a grader, and then stir your shredded cucumber, garlic, and yogurt together to make a tzatziki sauce. Slice the remaining cucumber into slices that are a quarter of an inch thick before placing them to the side.
4. Toast your pita bread, and then assemble your sandwich with each one having a tomato slice, a

few slices of cucumber, chickpea patty, and drizzle each one with your sauce to serve.

Nutrition: Calories: 387; Fat: 7g; Protein: 11g

Mushrooms with Soy Sauce Glaze

Preparation: 11 min | Cooking: 28 min | Servings: 2

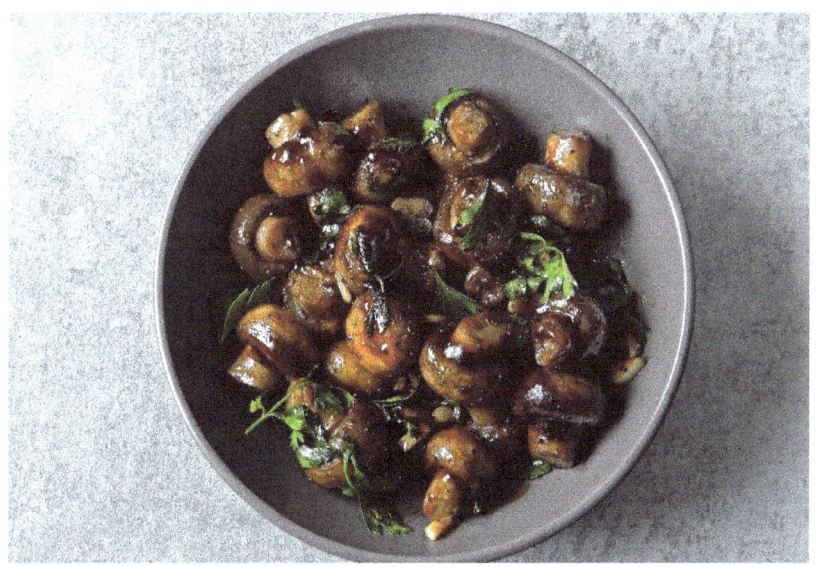

Ingredients

- 2 tablespoons butter
- 1 (8 oz.) package sliced white mushrooms
- 2 cloves garlic, minced
- 2 teaspoons soy sauce
- ground black pepper to taste

Directions

1. Undo the butter in a skillet; add the mushrooms; cook and stir until the mushrooms are soft and released about 5 min.
2. Stir in the garlic; keep cooking and stir for 1 minute. Pour the soy sauce; cook the mushrooms in the soy sauce until the liquid has evaporated, about 4 min.

Nutrition: Calories: 455; Fat: 11g; Protein: 18g

Cinnamon Quinoa Bars

Servings: 4 | Cooking: 30 min

Ingredients

- 2 ½ cups cooked quinoa
- 4 large eggs
- 1/3 cup unsweetened almond milk
- 1/3 cup pure maple syrup
- Seeds from ½ whole vanilla bean pod or 1 tbsp vanilla extract
- 1 ½ tbsp cinnamon
- 1/4 tsp salt

Directions

1. Preheat oven to 375oF.
2. Combine all ingredients into large bowl and mix well.
3. In an 8 x 8 Baking pan, cover with parchment paper.
4. Pour batter evenly into baking dish.
5. Bake for 25-30 minutes or until it has set. It should not wiggle when you lightly shake the pan because the eggs are fully cooked.

6. Remove as quickly as possible from pan and parchment paper onto cooling rack.
7. Cut into 4 pieces.
8. Enjoy on its own, with a small spread of almond or nut butter or wait until it cools to enjoy the next morning.

Nutrition: Calories per serving: 285; Carbs: 46.2g; Protein: 8.5g; Fat: 7.4g

Cucumber Olive Rice

Servings: 8 | Cooking: 10 min

Ingredients

- 2 cups rice, rinsed
- 1/2 cup olives, pitted
- 1 cup cucumber, chopped
- 1 tbsp red wine vinegar
- 1 tsp lemon zest, grated
- 1 tbsp fresh lemon juice
- 2 tbsp olive oil
- 2 cups vegetable broth
- 1/2 tsp dried oregano
- 1 red bell pepper, chopped
- 1/2 cup onion, chopped
- 1 tbsp olive oil
- Pepper
- Salt

Directions

1. Add oil into the inner pot of instant pot and set the pot on sauté mode.
2. Add onion and sauté for 3 minutes.

3. Add bell pepper and oregano and sauté for 1 minute.
4. Add rice and broth and stir well.
5. Seal pot with lid and cook on high for 6 minutes.
6. Once done, allow to release pressure naturally for 10 minutes then release remaining using quick release. Remove lid.
7. Add remaining ingredients and stir everything well to mix.
8. Serve immediately and enjoy it.

Nutrition: Calories 229 Fat 5.1 g Carbohydrates 40.2 g Sugar 1.6 g Protein 4.9 g Cholesterol 0 mg

Chicken And White Bean

Servings: 8 | Cooking: 70 min

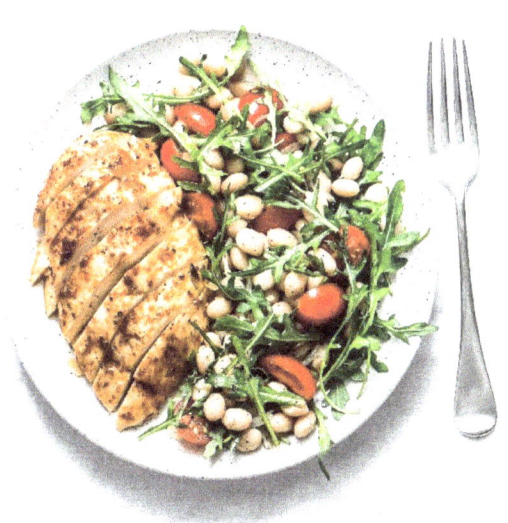

Ingredients

- 2 tbsp fresh cilantro, chopped
- 2 cups grated Monterey Jack cheese
- 3 cups water
- 1/8 tsp cayenne pepper
- 2 tsp pure chile powder
- 2 tsp ground cumin
- 1 4-oz can chopped green chiles

- 1 cup corn kernels
- 2 15-oz cans shite beans, drained and rinsed
- 2 garlic cloves
- 1 medium onion, diced
- 2 tbsp extra virgin olive oil
- 1 lb. chicken breasts, boneless and skinless

Directions

1. Slice chicken breasts into ½-inch cubes and with pepper and salt, season it.
2. On high fire, place a large nonstick fry pan and heat oil.
3. Sauté chicken pieces for three to four minutes or until lightly browned.
4. Reduce fire to medium and add garlic and onion.
5. Cook for 5 to 6 minutes or until onions are translucent.
6. Add water, spices, chilies, corn and beans. Bring to a boil.
7. Once boiling, slow fire to a simmer and continue simmering for an hour, uncovered.
8. To serve, garnish with a sprinkling of cilantro and a tablespoon of cheese.

Nutrition: Calories per serving: 433; Protein: 30.6g; Carbs: 29.5g; Fat: 21.8g

Chorizo-kidney Beans Quinoa Pilaf

Servings: 4 | Cooking: 35 min

Ingredients

- ¼ pound dried Spanish chorizo diced (about 2/3 cup)
- ¼ teaspoon red pepper flakes
- ¼ teaspoon smoked paprika
- ½ teaspoon cumin
- ½ teaspoon sea salt
- 1 3/4 cups water
- 1 cup quinoa
- 1 large clove garlic minced
- 1 small red bell pepper finely diced
- 1 small red onion finely diced
- 1 tablespoon tomato paste
- 1 15-ounce can kidney beans rinsed and drained

Directions

1. Place a nonstick pot on medium high fire and heat for 2 minutes. Add chorizo and sauté for 5 minutes until lightly browned.
2. Stir in peppers and onion. Sauté for 5 minutes.

3. Add tomato paste, red pepper flakes, salt, paprika, cumin, and garlic. Sauté for 2 minutes.
4. Stir in quinoa and mix well. Sauté for 2 minutes.
5. Add water and beans. Mix well. Cover and simmer for 20 minutes or until liquid is fully absorbed.
6. Turn off fire and fluff quinoa. Let it sit for 5 minutes more while uncovered.
7. Serve and enjoy.

Nutrition: Calories per serving: 260; Protein: 9.6g; Carbs: 40.9g; Fat: 6.8g

Belly-filling Cajun Rice & Chicken

Servings: 6 | Cooking: 20 min

Ingredients
- 1 tablespoon oil
- 1 onion, diced
- 3 cloves of garlic, minced
- 1-pound chicken breasts, sliced
- 1 tablespoon Cajun seasoning
- 1 tablespoon tomato paste
- 2 cups chicken broth
- 1 ½ cups white rice, rinsed
- 1 bell pepper, chopped

Directions
1. Press the Sauté on the Instant Pot and pour the oil.
2. Sauté the onion and garlic until fragrant.
3. Stir in the chicken breasts and season with Cajun seasoning.
4. Continue cooking for 3 minutes.
5. Add the tomato paste and chicken broth. Dissolve the tomato paste before adding the rice and bell pepper.

6. Close the lid and press the rice button.
7. Once done cooking, do a natural release for 10 minutes.
8. Then, do a quick release.
9. Once cooled, evenly divide into serving size, keep in your preferred container, and refrigerate until ready to eat.

Nutrition: Calories per serving: 337; Carbohydrates: 44.3g; Protein: 26.1g; Fat: 5.0g

Chapter 7: Dessert Recipes

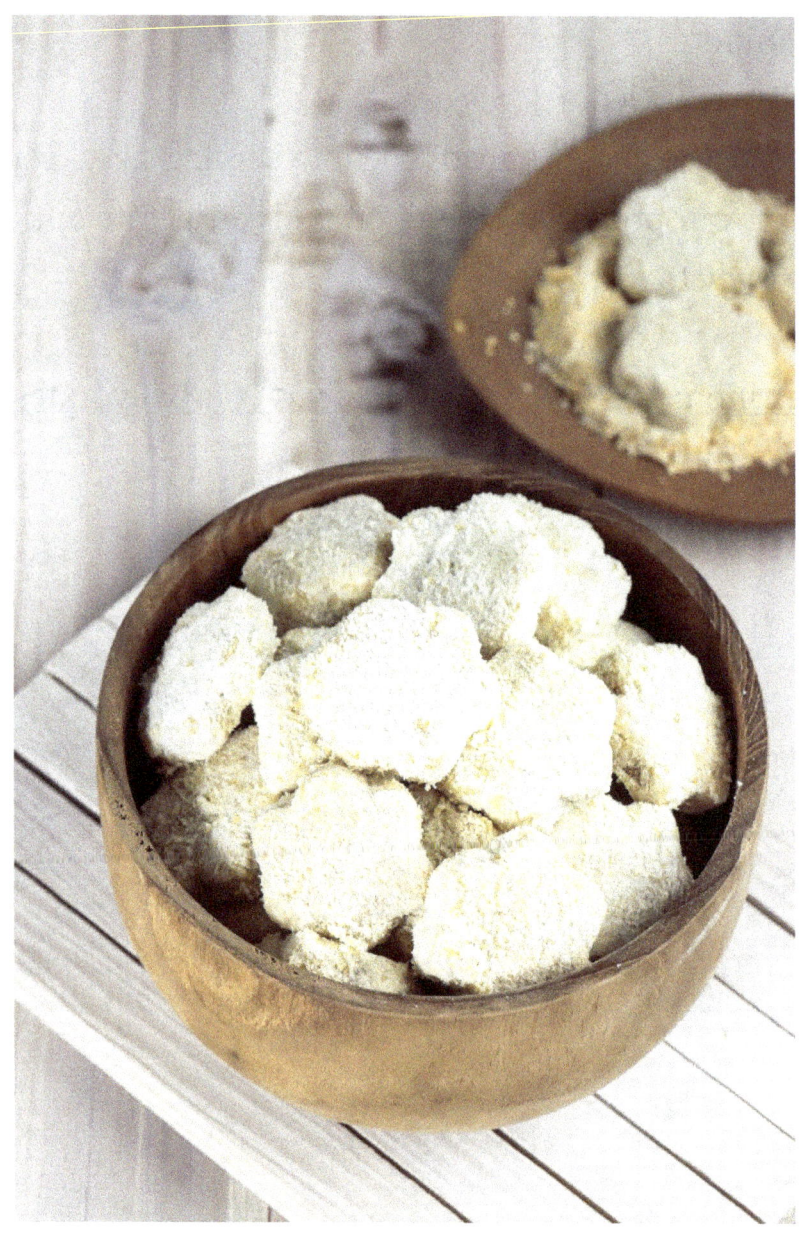

Almonds And Oats Pudding

Servings: 4 | Cooking: 15 min

Ingredients

- 1 tablespoon lemon juice
- Zest of 1 lime
- 1 and ½ cups almond milk
- 1 teaspoon almond extract
- ½ cup oats
- 2 tablespoons stevia
- ½ cup silver almonds, chopped

Directions

1. In a pan, combine the almond milk with the lime zest and the other ingredients, whisk, bring to a simmer and cook over medium heat for 15 minutes.
2. Divide the mix into bowls and serve cold.

Nutrition: calories 174; fat 12.1; fiber 3.2; carbs 3.9; protein 4.8

Chocolate Rice

Servings: 4 | Cooking: 20 min

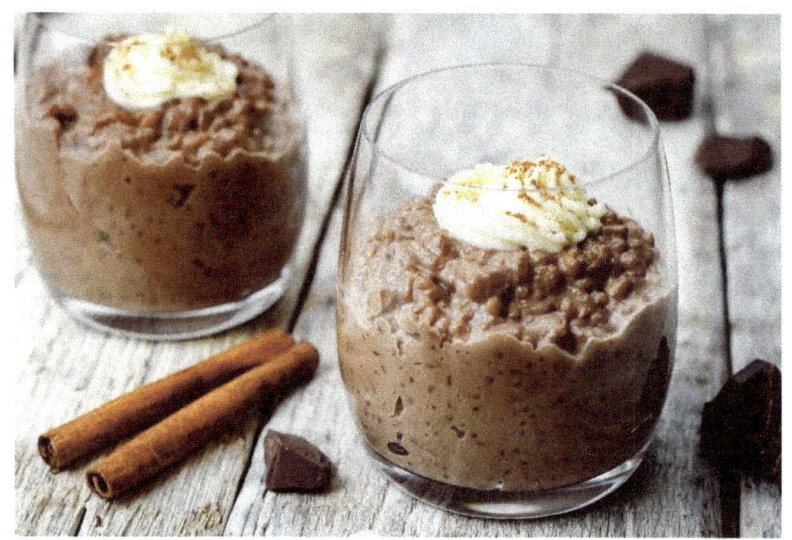

Ingredients

- 1 cup of rice
- 1 tbsp cocoa powder
- 2 tbsp maple syrup
- 2 cups almond milk

Directions

1. Add all ingredients into the inner pot of instant pot and stir well.
2. Seal pot with lid and cook on high for 20 minutes.

3. Once done, allow to release pressure naturally for 10 minutes then release remaining using quick release. Remove lid.
4. Stir and serve.

Nutrition: Calories 474 Fat 29.1 g Carbohydrates 51.1 g Sugar 10 g Protein 6.3 g Cholesterol 0 mg

Lemon And Semolina Cookies

Servings: 6 | Cooking: 20 min

Ingredients
- ½ teaspoon lemon zest, grated
- 4 tablespoons Erythritol
- 4 tablespoons semolina
- 2 tablespoons olive oil
- 8 tablespoons wheat flour, whole grain
- 1 teaspoon vanilla extract
- ½ teaspoon ground clove
- 3 tablespoons coconut oil
- ¼ teaspoon baking powder
- ¼ cup of water

Directions
1. Make the dough: in the mixing bowl combine together lemon zest, semolina, olive oil, wheat flour, vanilla extract, ground clove, coconut oil, and baking powder.
2. Knead the soft dough.
3. Make the small cookies in the shape of walnuts and press them gently with the help of the fork.

4. Line the baking tray with the baking paper.
5. Place the cookies in the tray and bake them for 20 minutes at 375F.
6. Meanwhile, bring the water to boil.
7. Add Erythritol and simmer the liquid for 2 minutes over the medium heat. Cool it.
8. Pour the cooled sweet water over the hot baked cookies and leave them for 10 minutes.
9. When the cookies soak all liquid, transfer them in the serving plates.

Nutrition: calories 165; fat 11.7; fiber 0.6; carbs 23.7; protein 2

Strawberry Sorbet

Servings: 2 | Cooking: 20 min

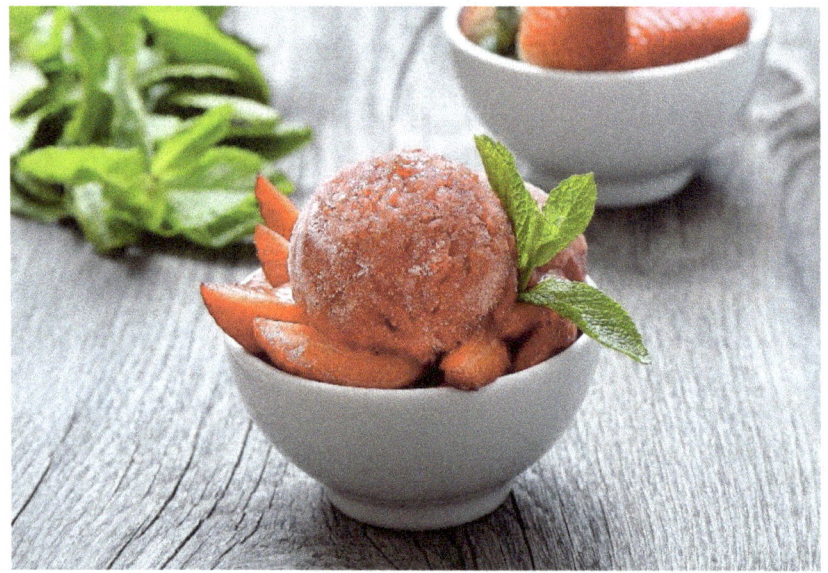

Ingredients

- 1 cup strawberries, chopped
- 1 tablespoon of liquid honey
- 2 tablespoons water
- 1 tablespoon lemon juice

Directions

1. Preheat the water and liquid honey until you get homogenous liquid.

2. Blend the strawberries until smooth and combine them with honey liquid and lemon juice.
3. Transfer the strawberry mixture in the ice cream maker and churn it for 20 minutes or until the sorbet is thick.
4. Scoop the cooked sorbet in the ice cream cups.

Nutrition: calories 57; fat 0.3; fiber 1.5; carbs 14.3; protein 0.6

Halva (halawa)

Servings: ¼ Cup | Cooking: 10 min

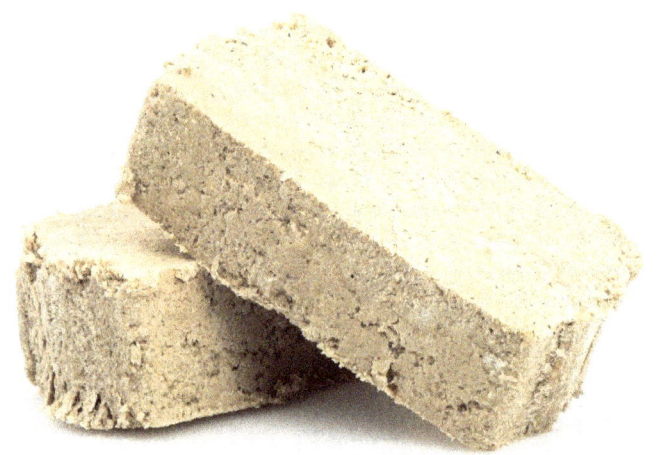

Ingredients

- 1 1/2 cups honey
- 1 1/2 cups tahini paste
- 1 cup pistachios, coarsely chopped

Directions

1. Pour honey into a saucepan, set over low heat, and bring to 240°F.

2. In another saucepan over low heat, bring tahini paste to 120°F.
3. In a bowl, whisk together heated honey and tahini paste until smooth. Fold in pistachios.
4. Line a loaf pan with parchment paper and spray with cooking spray. Pour tahini mixture into the loaf pan, and refrigerate for 2 days to set.
5. Cut halva into bite-size pieces, and serve.

CPSIA information can be obtained
at www.ICGtesting.com
Printed in the USA
BVHW011041160621
609723BV00013B/256